MW00345467

Professor Grow's
Book of Strains

The 50 Cannabis Strains Most Commonly Found at Dispensaries

The information contained in this book is not intended to diagnose, treat, cure or prevent any disease. Be sure to check with your health care practitioner before using medical marijuana.

Medical Marijuana use is NOT approved in all states. The information contained in this book is for patients and caregivers who are operating within their state and local laws. We do not advocate unlawful use of cannabis. Marijuana remains illegal under Federal Law. Use of marijuana, even for medical purposes carries a potential risk of arrest.

Be sure to review your local laws and obtain necessary permits before using medical marijuana.

Professor Grow's
Book of Strains

The 50 Cannabis Strains Most Commonly Found at Dispensaries

Justin Griswell and Victoria Young

Professor Grow's Book of Strains
Copyright © 2011 by Justin Griswell and Victoria Young
ISBN-13: 978-0615492032
ISBN-10: 0615492037

All rights reserved. No part of this book may be
reproduced in any form without written permission.

For information, contact:

Professor Grow, LLC
P. O. Box 366
Firestone, CO 80520-0366
professorgrow@gmail.com

Published by Professor Grow, LLC
Printed in the United States of America
First Edition: March 2011

Book Design by Victoria Young
"*Periodic Table of Cannabis*" and
Cover design by:
Victoria Young and Justin Griswell

This book is also available on Kindle.

Visit us online at: http://professorgrow.com

eMail us at: professorgrow@gmail.com.

Watch for our forthcoming books and classes on
Organic Gardening, Bonsai and Growing Medical Marijuana.

For Brother Duke and Pat....

And everyone
who is struggling with pain,
illness and depression.

Foreword

Professor Grow's Book of Strains grew organically out of the lives of the two authors. It was a natural progression of circumstances.

Victoria Young was diagnosed with an inherited neuromuscular disease in 1990. The symptoms include muscle wasting and severe nerve pain. Traditional medicine offered drugs that made her uncomfortable at best and very sick at worst. Drugs that were strong enough to help her sleep, left her drowsy, lethargic and unable to be productive. Other drugs caused extreme nausea to the point that she could not do anything at all.

Victoria resolved to find more natural ways to deal with pain. She altered her diet to eliminate or reduce allergens such as wheat, soy and dairy. It helped a little, but the pain was still there. She still had shooting pains that came without warning. Meditation helped a little, too.

Over time and with practice she was able to "ignore" the pain during the day when she was engaged in projects or something that could occupy her attention. The pain was still there, but she could put it on the "back burner" so-to-speak. Having her mind actively engaged in something took her mind off the pain.

But night was a different story. In order to get to sleep, she needed to "shut down" her mind. When she began to shut down her mind for sleep, all that was left was the pain.

Eventually, after several people suggested it, she got a doctor's recommendation to use marijuana and registered with the state, getting a card that enabled her to visit dispensaries and purchase cannabis. She was quite surprised at how well it helped her sleep. And she had no "hangover" the next day. It was welcome relief that she used only at night. There were some strains that caused a headache so she had to spend time trying strains to see which ones she tolerated well.

Her lungs could not tolerate smoke so she made brownies (wheat-free). It requires significantly more cannabis to make edibles than to smoke it for effect. And prices in the dispensaries were averaging $400 per ounce. Her best alternative became to grow her own medicine. Colorado, the state in which she resides, allows her to grow up to six plants at a time. A maximum of three can be flowering at one time.

Justin Griswell is Victoria's son. He is her designated caregiver registered with the state of Colorado. He had been growing and selling Bonsai trees for more than a dozen years. He also grows organic gardens and is very active with cultivating trees flowers and food. His knowledge of plants, growing nutrients and light is extensive.

Justin had studied many books and articles on growing cannabis and was able to put his considerable knowledge to work and assist Victoria in growing her own medicine.

During many months of experimentation with three plants at a time, they tried growing in soil and hydroponics. They eventually built their own grow lights, built their own hydroponics system and built their own screens to reflect and control light.

Their grow lights are NOT the typical HID lights that burn very hot and require great care and ventilation. Their CFL grow lights provide plenty of light (800 watts equivalent) for 3 plants and produce a nice yield. They do not require ventilation or heat mitigation. They designed and built a 6500k version for the vegetative state and a 2700k version for flowering.

Their homemade hydroponics system accommodates three plants nicely and produces a decent yield. They can harvest three plants every two to three months and stay within the state guidelines. Justin became inspired at the idea of helping patients (many of whom are disabled and on limited incomes) grow their own medicine safely and inexpensively (compared to dispensary prices).

During this process Justin and Victoria met other MMj patients who had dozens of questions about growing. Justin answered all of their questions with good, solid, easy-to-understand information. As a result, one of those people suggested that Justin call himself "Professor Grow" and teach this to others.

Victoria is in the domain name business so she quickly registered professorgrow.com and they began the process of developing Professor Grow LLC. Their mission is to teach growing classes, write books and create inexpensive "grow kits" that will enable patients and caregivers grow cannabis as medicine safely, inexpensively and easily within the laws of their individual states.

This book is the first in a series that we hope will help people figure out how to choose their strains and grow them as medicine where it is allowable by law.

__Preface__

We were already working on another book about growing and on outlines and PowerPoint presentations for growing classes when the idea for this book intervened.

I (Victoria) was still seeking ideal strains to treat my nerve pain so I could sleep at night. I wanted to identify up to 5 strains that worked well for me without side effects. I wanted to have other strains to switch to if my body built up a tolerance to one strain and it stopped working well.

The dispensaries kept guiding me to indica dominant strains and I kept getting headaches from most of them. Justin and I are still pondering whether it was the actual strains themselves, or perhaps some chemicals used in their growing. (Another reason to grow my own – we grow organically, whether it is food or medicine.)

I was trying to do some more research on strains without having to buy and try a sample of every strain available. My research included reading the descriptions dispensaries posted on websites. I found the descriptions to be pure marketing speak. No information in the description was related to what I wanted to know. The description would tell me how it looked, how it tasted and how much of a buzz I would get.

I wanted to know if it was supposed to be good for nerve pain, if it would help me sleep and if I would have lasting effects that would impair me in the morning. If I encountered a day in which I needed to use MMj in the daytime, I wanted a strain that would not give me "couchlock." And I needed to make sure any daytime strain I occasionally used would not interfere with my ability to focus and be productive. I did not want to be sitting at the computer with no ability to concentrate on what I was doing. I know from my own experience that some strains enable focus and some strains impair concentration.

Other research on the internet produced unsatisfactory results, as well. The myriad of "stoner forums" carried reviews (I use the term loosely) related to how messed up someone could get using it. They used strings of profanity to describe how totally stoned they became. (And they wonder why the mainstream hasn't accepted cannabis.) There were a few posts on some forums that gave some relevant information, but they were few and far between.

I told Justin that I wish we had the information that was valuable to me gathered up in one place. As we discussed it, we decided that it would be helpful for many Medical Marijuana users. Thus, The Book of Strains was born.

There are places on the internet that say there are over 1000 strains of cannabis. We decided to concentrate on the 50 strains that we most commonly see in dispensaries. Since we are in Colorado, we polled Colorado dispensaries. We also looked at the strain menus of many dispensaries in California. Although new strains may develop and popularity of some strains may wane, we believe these 50 strains represent the strains (and clones) that are most commonly available to MMj patients who visit dispensaries.

We plan to publish revised editions of this book when it is necessary to remain accurate and relevant.

DISCLAIMER: The information contained in this book is not intended to diagnose, treat, cure, or prevent any disease. Be sure to check with your health care practitioner before using medical marijuana.

Medical Marijuana use is NOT approved in all states. The information contained in this book is for patients and caregivers who are operating within their state and local laws. We do not advocate unlawful use of cannabis. Be sure to review your local laws, and obtain necessary permits before using medical marijuana. Use of marijuana, even for medicinal purposes, remains illegal under Federal law.

Introduction

We wrote this book to help MMj patients make more informed choices when going to a dispensary or choosing what to grow. We wanted to gather available information in one easy reference for Medical Marijuana Patients and Caregivers. The information contained herein is on the 50 Cannabis Strains most commonly found in dispensaries. We know these are the 50 strains to which most patients will have access in usable form(s) and as clones to grow.

When we started, we were open to covering as many strains as necessary in order to cover the most commonly available cannabis strains. Our research produced 50 strains that are the most commonly available in dispensaries, in usable form and/or clones.

We have organized the information with a two-page spread for each strain that contains relevant information for patients and caregivers. We have also provided indices that sort the information by the diseases for which people seek relief using cannabis.

And there is an index listing the current Medical Marijuana states and the diseases for which each state has approved MMj. Another index lists testing labs where you can get your strain(s) tested for cannabinoid content.

We recommend that you take some time to figure out what strains work best for you before you begin to grow. Visit a reputable dispensary or licensed caregiver or licensed grower to try small amounts of strains (buy only a gram of a new strain) to find out what will work for you. It is unnecessary out a significant amount of money to find out a strain doesn't work for your needs.

There are some <u>notable limitations</u> in this book:

- We cover only 50 strains out of over 1000 that are purported exist.

In our research we found that only 50 strains are very common in dispensaries. Individual dispensaries may carry a strain not found in this book, but it is not widely found at many dispensaries. We made the conscious decision to limit the scope of this book to the strains that one would most often find at a dispensary.

- None of the information in this book is intended to replace the advice of your licensed medical practitioner nor is it intended to diagnose, treat, cure or prevent any disease. Check with your licensed medical practitioner before using medical marijuana.

- We cannot guarantee the THC content of any strain. Our sources for info on THC content and genetics are seed banks' published strain info on the internet and information acquired from dispensaries, and published strain testing results from Full Spectrum Labs (http://fullspectrumlabs.com/tested/products/). We believe the THC info is reliable but cannot guarantee its accuracy. THC Content in one strain can vary dramatically due to differences in growing environments and growing methods. The only accurate way to ascertain true THC content is by having a sample tested by a lab. You can also ask your dispensary if they have had their strain(s) tested by a lab, and what the results were.

- There are multiple strains with the same name or multiple versions of some strains. We have seen AK-47 listed as 80% sativa at one dispensary and as 65% sativa at another. We have also seen Jilly Bean listed as 80% Indica in one dispensary and as 80% Sativa in another. In case of discrepancies we, looked at multiple sources and used the most prevalent response. We believe our information is accurate, but cannot guarantee the accuracy of Sativa/Indica content.

- We cannot guarantee that the strain of usable medicine clones or seeds you acquire are really the strain they are purported to be. There could be errors in labeling etc. We believe the majority of dispensaries and other licensed MMj outlets are carefully tracking their product (required in Colorado) so you should be able to rely on their statements but we cannot be responsible for any errors (they are human, after all) that your source may make.

- You cannot always know if a strain is pure or stable. Especially if you are acquiring your seeds or clones from an individual grower. We have seen cases where a patient acquired a clone of Hash Plant that was in no way similar to a Hash Plant clone acquired elsewhere. One of them could have been a cross or an unstable strain of Hash Plant that caused it to have different traits altogether.

- Medical Marijuana Laws in states including approved ailments and rules on growing are constantly changing. Info that was accurate at time of printing this book may be out-of-date when you read it. We will revise the book periodically but due to changes in laws and regulations beyond our control you should check with your state and local government agencies for current information on Medical Marijuana use in your area.

- This book is not for recreational cannabis users or for anyone who intends unlawful use of cannabis. We are providing this information as a service to medical marijuana patients and caregivers.

About Sativas and Indicas

When you are choosing your strain(s), there are a few generalities that are usually true about Sativas and Indicas. Keep in mind that each person's reaction to a particular strain can be quite different than the "norm," depending on the individual's circumstances.

Growing

Indicas tend to grow shorter (usually under 6 feet), bushier and have a shorter flowering time. Their leaves are more broad and full and deep green, sometimes with a purple tinge. Indicas tend to have more bud sites and usually produce smaller buds than Sativas. Indicas are usually more suited to indoor growing because of their shorter stature.

Sativas tend to grow tall (most are 8 to 12 feet, but some can grow to 25 feet), they have a longer flowering time and usually produce long buds. Most Sativas are more suited to outdoor growing because of their sheer size. However, some breeders have developed Sativa dominant strains that grow more like an Indica.

Body Effects

Indicas have more full body effects and are touted for pain, insomnia, loss of appetite, etc. They are more often consumed at night, when getting ready for sleep.

Sativas have a more cerebral effect. They can improve mood, give a feeling of optimism and well-being, as well as some pain relief. Sativas are often recommended for depression, anxiety, increasing creativity, and are usually consumed during the day time.

TABLE OF CONTENTS

TABLE OF CONTENTS

TABLE OF CONTENTS

TABLE OF CONTENTS

The Strains

<u>Afghan Goo (aka Afghooey)</u>

Lineage: Maui Haze X Afghani #1

Genetics: 80% (I) — 20% (S)

THC Content: 16% — 20%

Past Medicinal Uses*:

AIDS
Alcoholism
Anorexia
Anxiety
Appetite
Arthritis
Cancer
Depression
Epilepsy
Gastrointestinal Issues
Glaucoma
Insomnia
Migraines
MS
Muscle Spasms
Nausea
Pain
PMS
PTSD

```
        ┌─────────────┐
        │          Ih │
        │             │
        │   Ag        │
        │  80/20      │
        └─────────────┘
```

Growing: Easy

Flowering Time: 60-65 Days

Description: This strain doesn't get very tall. Its short stature makes it a good candidate for growing in small places.

It is a good plant to top two or three times during the vegetative stage to produce more budding sites. You can find out more about topping your plants by visiting:

http://professorgrow.com/2010/09/21/mmj-corner-topping-and-cropping-to-increase-your-yield/

Afghan Goo could be a good strain for a beginning grower, because it is an easy plant to manage in small spaces.

*The _**Past Medicinal Uses**_ information in this book is NOT intended to replace the advice of your licensed medical practitioner nor is it intended to diagnose, treat, cure or prevent any disease. It is merely a listing of some historical uses for this particular strain. Contact your licensed medical professional for advice on using various strains for your ailments.

<u>Afghooey Train Wreck</u>

Lineage: Afghani X Columbian X Mexican

Genetics: 50% (S) 50% (I)

THC Content: 15% — 20%

Past Medicinal Uses*:

Appetite Stimulation

Cramps

Depression

Fibromyalgia

Joint Pain

Migraines

Muscle Pain

Nausea

Pain Relief

	H
At	
50/50	

Growing: Easy

Flowering: 42 - 67 Days

Description: This strain is a 50/50 mix. We would suggest topping the plant three to four times during the vegetative stage. (For information on topping plants, visit http://professorgrow.com.) This is because of the possible height the plant may get.

Afghooey Train Wreck takes after its Sativa genetics in the height department. Topping helps keep the height under control and bush the plant out a bit. This can be a good candidate for smaller indoor grow spaces, since this strain is a 50-50 mix. The flowering period will vary if you are growing from seeds. If you are growing from clones then you will have a more uniform growing and flowering.

We recommend growing this strain from clones.

*The **_Past Medicinal Uses_** information in this book is NOT intended to replace the advice of your licensed medical practitioner nor is it intended to diagnose, treat, cure or prevent any disease. It is merely a listing of some historical uses for this particular strain. Contact your licensed medical professional for advice on using various strains for your ailments.

<u>AK-47</u>

Lineage: Columbian, Mexican X Thai, Afghani

Genetics: 65% (S) 35% (I)

THC Content: 18% — 20%

Awards: 1999 Sativa Cup 2nd Place

Past Medicinal Uses*:

Alzheimer's Disease

Bipolar Disorder

Chronic Pain

Depression

Headache

Nausea

Poor Appetite

Vomiting

Sh

Ak₄₇

65/35

Growing: Moderate

Flowering: 60 - 75 Days

Description: This strain is a Sativa dominant. It tends to grow tall. We would suggest topping the plant three to four times during the vegetative stage because of limited side branching.

You can find out more about topping your plants by visiting:

http://professorgrow.com/2010/09/21/mmj-corner-topping-and-cropping-to-increase-your-yield/

This plant will need a little more room to grow. When putting in to your grow room keep this in mind. If you have a small grow room, we suggest you only grow two plants because of height, and lengthy flowering time.

*The _**Past Medicinal Uses**_ information in this book is NOT intended to replace the advice of your licensed medical practitioner nor is it intended to diagnose, treat, cure or prevent any disease. It is merely a listing of some historical uses for this particular strain. Contact your licensed medical professional for advice on using various strains for your ailments.

Banana Kush

Lineage: OG Kush X Banana

Genetics: 60% (I) 40% (S)

THC Content: 18% — 20%

Past Medicinal Uses*:

Eating Disorders

Fibromyalgia

Glaucoma

Insomnia

Joint Pain

Muscle Spasms

Nausea

Pain Relief

Phantom Limb Pain

```
┌─────────────┐
│          Ih │
│   Bk        │
│   60/40     │
└─────────────┘
```

Growing: Moderate

Flowering: 55 - 60 Days

Description: This strain is an Indica dominant. It won't get very tall. We suggest topping it three to four times during the vegetative stage to produce more budding sites. Banana Kush is a good candidate for small grow rooms, because of its shorter stature.

You can find out more about topping your plants by visiting:

http://professorgrow.com/2010/09/21/mmj-corner-topping-and-cropping-to-increase-your-yield/

Just keep a good eye on the plant during the flowering period. The flowers tend to grow very close to the main stock.

*The **_Past Medicinal Uses_** information in this book is NOT intended to replace the advice of your licensed medical practitioner nor is it intended to diagnose, treat, cure or prevent any disease. It is merely a listing of some historical uses for this particular strain. Contact your licensed medical professional for advice on using various strains for your ailments.

<u>Big Bud</u>

Lineage: Skunk,Big Bud X NL#5

Genetics: 75% (I) 25% (S)

THC Content: 8% — 15%

Past Medicinal Uses*:

Anxiety

Appetite

Depression

Insomnia

Migraines

MS

Nausea

Stomach Pains

Stress

Tourette's Syndrome

```
                    Ih
        Bb
        75/25
```

Growing: Easy

Flowering: 60 - 74 Days

Description: This is a great Indica dominant strain to grow in a small room, and produce good medicine yields. This plant won't get very tall during vegetative stage. During flowering stage you will want to give the plant plenty of room to produce its large buds. We would suggest to only grow two plants in a small grow room with the amount of medicine you produce. This plant has great natural side branching, so we would only suggest topping two to three times in a small grow room. You can find out more about topping your plants by visiting:

http://professorgrow.com/2010/09/21/mmj-corner-topping-and-cropping-to-increase-your-yield/

If you want more side branching, you can top it more if you have a larger grow area.

*The **_Past Medicinal Uses_** information in this book is NOT intended to replace the advice of your licensed medical practitioner nor is it intended to diagnose, treat, cure or prevent any disease. It is merely a listing of some historical uses for this particular strain. Contact your licensed medical professional for advice on using various strains for your ailments.

Blue Dream

Lineage: Blueberry X Haze

Genetics: 80% (S) 20% (I)

THC Content: 15% — 20%

Past Medicinal Uses*:

AIDS

Anorexia

Appetite

Arthritis

Cancer

Depression

Epilepsy

Gastrointestinal Issues

Glaucoma

MS

Muscle Spasms

Nausea

Pain Relief

PTSD

```
                    Sh
        Bd
       80/20
```

Growing: Moderate

Flowering: 60 - 70 Days

Description: This strain is a Sativa dominant. This strain can get very tall. We suggest topping four to five times during the vegetative stage in order to keep the height in a good level for the flowering stage. A good rule of thumb is that the pure Sativa and heavily Sativa dominant strains will double in height during flowering. So, if you put it into flowering at 3 feet tall, it will be about 6 feet tall at harvest time. Frequent topping produces more side branches and keeps height under control. Find out more about topping your plants by visiting: http://professorgrow.com/ and search on term "topping."

This is not a good strain for a small grow room, because of height and flowering time. You could grow one Blue Dream plant in a smaller grow room.

*The **_Past Medicinal Uses_** information in this book is NOT intended to replace the advice of your licensed medical practitioner nor is it intended to diagnose, treat, cure or prevent any disease. It is merely a listing of some historical uses for this particular strain. Contact your licensed medical professional for advice on using various strains for your ailments.

Blue Moonshine

Lineage: Highland Thai X Afghan

Genetics: 90% (I) 10% (S)

THC Content: 15% — 21%

Past Medicinal Uses*:

Anorexia

Anticonvulsant

Anxiety

Appetite Stimulation

Depression

Insomnia

Nausea

Pain Relief

Stress

Bm Ih
90/10

Growing: Easy

Flowering: 45 - 55 Days

Description: Blue Moonshine is almost a pure Indica. It tends to stay small. We would suggest topping the plant two to three times during the vegetative stage to create more budding sites. You can find out more about topping your plants by visiting:

http://professorgrow.com/2010/09/21/mmj-corner-topping-and-cropping-to-increase-your-yield/

Because of its short stature, Blue Moonshine is ideal for the small grow room. With heavy topping three plants will do well in a small grow room.

*The **_Past Medicinal Uses_** information in this book is NOT intended to replace the advice of your licensed medical practitioner nor is it intended to diagnose, treat, cure or prevent any disease. It is merely a listing of some historical uses for this particular strain. Contact your licensed medical professional for advice on using various strains for your ailments.

<u>Blueberry</u>

Lineage: Purple Thai X Afghan

Genetics: 80% (I) 20% (S)

THC Content: 15% — 21%

Awards: 2000 Cannabis Cup 1st Place
2000 Indica Cup 1st Place
2001 Cannabis Cup 2nd Place
2001 Indica Cup 3rd Place

Past Medicinal Uses*:

AIDS
Anorexia
Anxiety
Chronic Pain
Depressive Disorder
Diarrhea
Emotional Lability
Gastrointestinal Disorder
Insomnia
Muscle Pain
Muscle Spasm
Nausea
Pain

Ih

B

80/20

Growing: Easy

Flowering: 45 - 55 Days

Description: Blueberry is an Indica dominant strain. This strain does very well in small grow rooms. The plant tends to stay short. We would suggest topping the plant three to four times during the vegetative stage.

This will help produce more budding sites. You can find out more about topping your plants by visiting:

http://professorgrow.com/2010/09/21/mmj-corner-topping-and-cropping-to-increase-your-yield/

Blueberry has good side branching, so if you don't want top it, you will still produce a good amount of medicine.

*The ___Past Medicinal Uses___ information in this book is NOT intended to replace the advice of your licensed medical practitioner nor is it intended to diagnose, treat, cure or prevent any disease. It is merely a listing of some historical uses for this particular strain. Contact your licensed medical professional for advice on using various strains for your ailments.

Bubba Kush

Lineage: Bubble Gum X Kush

Genetics: 60% (I) 40% (S)

THC Content: 15% — 18%

Past Medicinal Uses*:

Aches

Anxiety

Headaches

Insomnia

Pain

Soreness

Stiff Muscles

```
         Ih
  Bbk
  60/40
```

Growing: Easy

Flowering: 60 - 70 Days

Description: Bubba Kush is an Indica dominant strain. It tends to grow to a medium height. We would suggest topping two to three times during the vegetative stage because of low side branching. You can find out more about topping your plants by visiting:

http://professorgrow.com/2010/09/21/mmj-corner-topping-and-cropping-to-increase-your-yield/

This is a good plant for a small grow room. Three plants would do well in a smaller growing area. Just keep in mind that Bubba Kush does have a little longer flowering period than most Indicas. Remember to top it a few times to increase side branching and increase bud sites for a better yield.

*The **_Past Medicinal Uses_** information in this book is NOT intended to replace the advice of your licensed medical practitioner nor is it intended to diagnose, treat, cure or prevent any disease. It is merely a listing of some historical uses for this particular strain. Contact your licensed medical professional for advice on using various strains for your ailments.

<u>Bubble Berry</u>

Lineage: Bubblegum X Blueberry

Genetics: 80% (S) 20% (I)

THC Content: 15% — 20%

Past Medicinal Uses*:

ADD

Depression

Epilepsy

Insomnia

Loss of Appetite

Migraines

Muscle Tension

Pain Relief

Stomach Ulcers

Stress

```
         ┌──────────────┐
         │           Sh │
         │    Bu        │
         │   80/20      │
         └──────────────┘
```

Growing: Easy

Flowering: 50 - 60 Days

Description: Bubble Berry is a Sativa dominant strain. It tends to grow to a medium height. The good thing about this strain is the shorter than usual flowering time for a Sativa dominant strain.

This strain can be grown in a small grow room. You probably should grow no more than two plants in a small growing area, due to the size of the Sativa strain.

We suggest that you top these plants three to four times during the vegetative cycle. You can find out more about topping your plants by visiting:

http://professorgrow.com/2010/09/21/mmj-corner-topping-and-cropping-to-increase-your-yield/

*The ***Past Medicinal Uses*** information in this book is NOT intended to replace the advice of your licensed medical practitioner nor is it intended to diagnose, treat, cure or prevent any disease. It is merely a listing of some historical uses for this particular strain. Contact your licensed medical professional for advice on using various strains for your ailments.

Bubble Gum

Lineage: Big Skunk X NL #5

Genetics: 60% (I) 40% (S)

THC Content: 15% — 20%

Awards: 1995 Cannabis Cup 2nd Place

Past Medicinal Uses*:

ADD

Alzheimer's Disease

Anticonvulsant

Anxiety

Appetite Stimulant

Depression

Glaucoma

Muscle Spasms

Nausea

Stress

```
        ┌─────────────┐
        │          Ih │
        │    Bg       │
        │   60/40     │
        └─────────────┘
```

Growing: Moderate

Flowering: 56 - 63 Days

Description: Bubble Gum is a Sativa dominant strain. It tends to grow tall. We would suggest topping the plant three to four times during the vegetative stage to keep it to a manageable height. For information on topping plants, visit:

http://professorgrow.com /2010/09/21/mmj-corner-topping-and-cropping-to-increase-your-yield/)

This plant will need a little more room to grow. When putting Bubble Gum into your grow room keep this in mind, especially if you have a small grow room. We suggest you only grow two plants because of the height, and flowering time of this strain.

*The _**Past Medicinal Uses**_ information in this book is NOT intended to replace the advice of your licensed medical practitioner nor is it intended to diagnose, treat, cure or prevent any disease. It is merely a listing of some historical uses for this particular strain. Contact your licensed medical professional for advice on using various strains for your ailments.

Buddha's Sister

Lineage: Reclining Buddha X Afghani Hawaiian

Genetics: 80% (I) 20% (S)

THC Content: 15% — 20%

Awards: 2002 Indica Cup 2nd Place

Past Medicinal Uses*:

ADD

ADHD

ALS

Appetite Stimulation

Body Aches

Depression

Epilepsy

Insomnia

Lou Gehrig's Disease

Nausea

```
        Ih
  Bs
 80/20
```

Growing: Moderate

Flowering: 67 - 75 Days

Description: Buddha's Sister is an Indica dominant strain. It tends to grow to a medium height. It also has good natural side branching.

Because of the natural side branching, you don't need to top this strain as much as others. You may still want to top it once or twice during the vegetative stage. Find out more about topping your plants by visiting:

http://professorgrow.com/2010/09/21/mmj-corner-topping-and-cropping-to-increase-your-yield/

Buddha's Sister has a longer flowing time than most plants with this much Indica in them, so keep that in mind if choosing to grow it. This is a good plant for a small grow room. Two to three plants will do well. Keep the side branching in mind when growing in a small grow room.

*The ***Past Medicinal Uses*** information in this book is NOT intended to replace the advice of your licensed medical practitioner nor is it intended to diagnose, treat, cure or prevent any disease. It is merely a listing of some historical uses for this particular strain. Contact your licensed medical professional for advice on using various strains for your ailments.

<u>Chem Dog</u> (aka Chem Dawg)

Lineage: OG Kush X Sour Diesel

Genetics: 60% (I) 40% (S)

THC Content: 15% — 20%

Past Medicinal Uses*:

Anxiety

Deep Muscle Pain

Glaucoma

Joint Pains

Mood Elevation

Movement Disorders

Nausea

Restless Behaviors

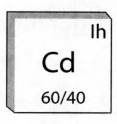

Growing: Easy-Moderate

Flowering: 60 - 70 Days

Description: Chem Dog is an Indica dominant strain. It tends to grow to a taller height than most Indicas.

We would suggest topping the plant three to four times during the vegetative stage. You can find out more about topping your plants by visiting:

http://professorgrow.com/2010/09/21/mmj-corner-topping-and-cropping-to-increase-your-yield/

This plant will need a little more room to grow. When putting Chem Dog into your grow room, keep this in mind, especially if you have a small grow room. We suggest you only grow two plants in a small grow room because of height, and flowering time.

*The _**Past Medicinal Uses**_ information in this book is NOT intended to replace the advice of your licensed medical practitioner nor is it intended to diagnose, treat, cure or prevent any disease. It is merely a listing of some historical uses for this particular strain. Contact your licensed medical professional for advice on using various strains for your ailments.

<u>Chocolope</u>

Lineage: O.G. Chocolate Thai X Cantaloupe Haze

Genetics: 100% (S)

THC Content: 15% — 20%

Awards: 2007 Cannabis Cup 2nd Place
2008 Cannabis Cup 3rd Place
2010 Sativa Cup 2nd Place

Past Medicinal Uses*:

Anorexia

Arthritis Pain

Cancer

Chronic Pain

Depression

Glaucoma

Headache

Migraines

Nausea

```
        S
  Ch
  100
```

Growing: Difficult

Flowering: 63 - 70 Days

Description: Chocolope is a pure Sativa strain. This plant will grow very tall. We would suggest topping the plant three to four times during the vegetative stage. You can find out more about topping your plants by visiting:

http://professorgrow.com/2010/09/21/mmj-corner-topping-and-cropping-to-increase-your-yield/

Also after two-to-two-and-a-half weeks in vegetative state (or when the plant is about 18 - 24 inches tall), change the light cycle to the flowering setting. The plant will continue to grow at least 12 to 18 inches in the flowering stage. Chocolope is not recommended for a small growing area.

*The ***Past Medicinal Uses*** information in this book is NOT intended to replace the advice of your licensed medical practitioner nor is it intended to diagnose, treat, cure or prevent any disease. It is merely a listing of some historical uses for this particular strain. Contact your licensed medical professional for advice on using various strains for your ailments.

<u>Durban Poison</u>

Lineage: South Africa Landrace Sativa

Genetics: 100% (S)

THC Content: 14% — 16%

Past Medicinal Uses*:

ADD

Anxiety

Appetite Stimulation

Cancer

Depression

Glaucoma

Inflammation

Joint Pain

Migraines

MS

Muscle Pain

Nausea

Neuropathic Pain

Phantom Limb Pain

Dp
S
100

Growing: Difficult

Flowering: 65 - 74 Days

Description: This a pure Sativa strain. This plant will grow very tall. We would suggest topping the plant three to four times during the vegetative stage.

You can find out more about topping your plants by visiting: http://professorgrow.com/2010/09/21/mmj-corner-topping-and-cropping-to-increase-your-yield/

Also after two-or-two-and-a-half weeks in vegetative state (or when the plant is 18-to-24 inches tall), change the light cycle to the flowering setting. The plant will continue to grow at least 12 to 18 inches in the flowering stage, perhaps more.

Durban Poison is not recommended for a small growing area.

*The ***Past Medicinal Uses*** information in this book is NOT intended to replace the advice of your licensed medical practitioner nor is it intended to diagnose, treat, cure or prevent any disease. It is merely a listing of some historical uses for this particular strain. Contact your licensed medical professional for advice on using various strains for your ailments.

<u>Flo</u>

Lineage: Purple Thai X Afghan Indica

Genetics: 60% (S) 40% (I)

THC Content: 15% — 20%

Past Medicinal Uses*:

Anti-Anxiety

Anti-Fatigue

Appetite Stimulation

Energy

Mood Elevation

Muscle Tension

Pain Relief

Relaxation

Strong Ocular Attention

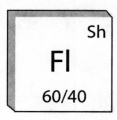

Growing: Moderate

Flowering: 50 - 55 Days

Description: This is a Sativa dominant strain, but the leaves and side-branching show off its Indica portion of the genetics. This plant tends to grow to a medium height. It also has good natural side branching.

This is a good plant for a small grow room. Two plants will do well. Just keep the side branching in mind when growing in a small grow room. It is a good plant to top two or three times to control the height. You can find out more about topping your plants by visiting:

http://professorgrow.com/2010/09/21/mmj-corner-topping-and-cropping-to-increase-your-yield/

*The ***Past Medicinal Uses*** information in this book is NOT intended to replace the advice of your licensed medical practitioner nor is it intended to diagnose, treat, cure or prevent any disease. It is merely a listing of some historical uses for this particular strain. Contact your licensed medical professional for advice on using various strains for your ailments.

G-13

Lineage: Afghani Descent

Genetics: 100% (I)

THC Content: 18% — 25%

Past Medicinal Uses*:

Arthritis

Cancer

Fibromyalgia

Glaucoma

HIV/AIDS

Inflammation

Joint Pain

Muscle Pain

Muscle Spasms

Nausea

Neuropathic Pain

Pain Killer

Skin Irritation

Growing: Easy

Flowering: 45 - 50 Days

Description: G-13 is a pure Indica strain. This plant tends to grow to a small-to-medium height. The G-13 plant doesn't produce any side branching. We would suggest topping this plant three to four times.

You can find out more about topping your plants by visiting:

http://professorgrow.com/2010/09/21/mmj-corner-topping-and-cropping-to-increase-your-yield/

This plant is good for a small grow room. Three plants could be grown well in a small grow area.

*The ***Past Medicinal Uses*** information in this book is NOT intended to replace the advice of your licensed medical practitioner nor is it intended to diagnose, treat, cure or prevent any disease. It is merely a listing of some historical uses for this particular strain. Contact your licensed medical professional for advice on using various strains for your ailments.

G-13 x Haze

Lineage: G-13 X Original Haze

Genetics: 80% (I) 20% (S)

THC Content: 18% — 20%

Awards: 2006 Cannabis Cup 2nd Place
2007 Cannabis Cup 1st Place

Past Medicinal Uses*:

ADD

ADHD

Anticonvulsant

Anxiety

Appetite Stimulation

Arthritis

Chronic Pain

Depression

Epilepsy

Gastrointestinal Disorder

Insomnia

Migraines

```
         lh
    Gh
    80/20
```

Growing: Moderate

Flowering: 55 - 70 Days

Description: G-13 crossed with Haze is an Indica dominant strain. It tends to grow to a medium height. It will have some side branching. We would still suggest to top the plant two to three times.

You can find out more about topping your plants by visiting:

http://professorgrow.com/2010/09/21/mmj-corner-topping-and-cropping-to-increase-your-yield/

This is a good plant for a small grow room. Two to three plants will do well. Keep in mind that it does have longer flowing time than most plants with this much Indica in them.

*The **_Past Medicinal Uses_** information in this book is NOT intended to replace the advice of your licensed medical practitioner nor is it intended to diagnose, treat, cure or prevent any disease. It is merely a listing of some historical uses for this particular strain. Contact your licensed medical professional for advice on using various strains for your ailments.

__Grand Daddy Purple__

Lineage: Purple Erkle X Big Bud

Genetics: 100% (I)

THC Content: 15% — 20%

Past Medicinal Uses*:

Appetite Stimulation

Insomnia

Joint Pain

Migraines

Nausea

Pain Relief

Relaxation

Gp
I
100

Growing: Easy

Flowering: 55 - 60 Days

Description: Grand Daddy Purple is a pure Indica strain. It tends to grow to a small-medium height. We would not suggest topping because of good natural side branching.

Because you don't have to spend time topping and otherwise controlling the height and shape of the plant, it is ideal for a beginning grower. The flowering time is shorter than many strains, as well.

This is a great plant for the small grow room. Three plants will do well in a small grow room.

*The **_Past Medicinal Uses_** information in this book is NOT intended to replace the advice of your licensed medical practitioner nor is it intended to diagnose, treat, cure or prevent any disease. It is merely a listing of some historical uses for this particular strain. Contact your licensed medical professional for advice on using various strains for your ailments.

<u>Grapefruit</u>

Lineage: C-99 X Fruity Sativa

Genetics: 80% (S) 20% (I)

THC Content: 15% — 20%

Past Medicinal Uses*:

Anti-Anxiety

Anti-Depression

Appetite Stimulation

Hypertension

Insomnia

Possible Ocular Relief

Relaxation

```
        ┌──────────┐
        │       Sh │
        │   Gf     │
        │  80/20   │
        └──────────┘
```

Growing: Easy-Moderate

Flowering: 50 - 55 Days

Description: Grapefruit is a Sativa dominant strain. It tends to grow to a small-medium height, shorter than most Sativa strains.

Like other Sativas, this is a fast growing plant. We would suggest topping the plant early on. Top it two to three times during the vegetative stage because of its fast growth. You can find out more about topping your plants by visiting:

http://professorgrow.com/2010/09/21/mmj-corner-topping-and-cropping-to-increase-your-yield/

This a good plant for a small grow room. Just keep an eye on it because of its quick growth, and fast flowering time.

*The **_Past Medicinal Uses_** information in this book is NOT intended to replace the advice of your licensed medical practitioner nor is it intended to diagnose, treat, cure or prevent any disease. It is merely a listing of some historical uses for this particular strain. Contact your licensed medical professional for advice on using various strains for your ailments.

Hash Plant

Lineage: Lebanese X Thai X Northern Lights #1

Genetics: 100% (I)

THC Content: 15% — 20%

Past Medicinal Uses*:

Anxiety

Appetite Stimulation

Bipolar Disorder

Chronic Pain

Depression

Headache

Migraines

Nausea

Nervousness

Relaxation

Stress

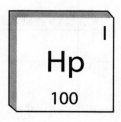

Hp

I

100

Growing: Easy

Flowering: 40 - 45 Days

Description: Hash Plant is a pure Indica strain. It tends to grow small with not much side branching.

We would suggest topping three to four times to let the plant bush out a little more, because of its short stature. Bushing it out will produce more budding sites when it goes into flowering. You can find out more about topping your plants by visiting:

http://professorgrow.com/2010/09/21/mmj-corner-topping-and-cropping-to-increase-your-yield/

This plant is ideal for the small grow room. With heavy topping three plants will do well in a small grow room.

*The _**Past Medicinal Uses**_ information in this book is NOT intended to replace the advice of your licensed medical practitioner nor is it intended to diagnose, treat, cure or prevent any disease. It is merely a listing of some historical uses for this particular strain. Contact your licensed medical professional for advice on using various strains for your ailments.

<u>Hawaiian</u>

Lineage: Hawaiian Landrace Sativa

Genetics: 100% (S)

THC Content: 15% — 20%

Past Medicinal Uses*:

Anxiety

Depression

Epilepsy

Glaucoma

Mood Elevation

Pain

Seizures

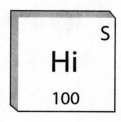

Growing: Difficult

Flowering: 86 - 100 Days

Description: Hawaiian a pure Sativa strain. This plant will grow very tall. It grows best outdoors where it has plenty of room.

We would suggest topping the plant three to four times during the vegetative stage. Find out more about topping your plants by visiting:

http://professorgrow.com/2010/09/21/mmj-corner-topping-and-cropping-to-increase-your-yield/

Because this plant grows so big, after two-to-two-and-a-half weeks in vegetative state (or when the plant reaches 18 to 24 inches tall), change the light cycle to the flowering setting. The plant will continue to grow at least 12 to 18 inches in the flowering stage. Hawaiian is not recommended for a small growing area.

*The ***Past Medicinal Uses*** information in this book is NOT intended to replace the advice of your licensed medical practitioner nor is it intended to diagnose, treat, cure or prevent any disease. It is merely a listing of some historical uses for this particular strain. Contact your licensed medical professional for advice on using various strains for your ailments.

Hawaiian Skunk

Lineage: Hawaiian X Skunk #1

Genetics: 60% (S) 40% (I)*

THC Content: 15% — 20%

Past Medicinal Uses*:

ADD

Anxiety

Appetite Stimulation

Depression

Insomnia

Migraines

Pain

Stress

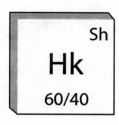

Growing: Moderate

Flowering: 68 - 80 Days

Description: Hawaiian Skunk is a Sativa dominant strain. It tends to grow tall.

We would suggest topping the plant three to four times during the vegetative stage. You can find out more about topping your plants by visiting:

http://professorgrow.com/2010/09/21/mmj-corner-topping-and-cropping-to-increase-your-yield/

This plant will need a little more room to grow. Keep this in mind if you have a small grow room. We suggest you only grow two plants because of height, and long flowering time.

*The **_Past Medicinal Uses_** information in this book is NOT intended to replace the advice of your licensed medical practitioner nor is it intended to diagnose, treat, cure or prevent any disease. It is merely a listing of some historical uses for this particular strain. Contact your licensed medical professional for advice on using various strains for your ailments.

<u>Hawaiian Snow</u>

Lineage: Hawaiian Haze X Pure Haze X Neville's Haze

Genetics: 90% (S) 10% (I)

THC Content: 15% — 23%

Awards: 2003 Cannabis Cup 1st Place
2003 Sativa Cup 3rd Place

Past Medicinal Uses*:

Depression

Glaucoma

Inflammation

Joint Pain

Migraines

Nausea

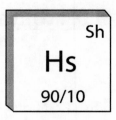

Growing: Difficult

Flowering: 105 - 112 Days

Description: Hawaiian Snow is almost a pure Sativa. This plant will grow very tall. We would suggest topping the plant three to four times during the vegetative stage. You can find out more about topping your plants by visiting:

http://professorgrow.com/2010/09/21/mmj-corner-topping-and-cropping-to-increase-your-yield/

 Also, after two-to-two-and-a-half weeks in vegetative state (or when the plant is 18-to-24 inches tall), change the light cycle to the flowering setting. The plant will continue to grow at least 12 to 18 inches in the flowering stage, perhaps more. Hawaiian Snow is not recommended for a small growing area.

*The _**Past Medicinal Uses**_ information in this book is NOT intended to replace the advice of your licensed medical practitioner nor is it intended to diagnose, treat, cure or prevent any disease. It is merely a listing of some historical uses for this particular strain. Contact your licensed medical professional for advice on using various strains for your ailments.

<u>Headband</u>

Lineage: OG Kush X Master Kush X Sour Diesel]

Genetics: 85% (I) 15% (S)

THC Content: 15% — 20%

Awards: 2009 Cannabis Cup 3rd Place

Past Medicinal Uses*:

ADD

AIDS

Anorexia

Arthritis

Cancer

Depression

Epilepsy

Glaucoma

Migraines

Multiple Sclerosis

Muscle Spasms

Nausea

Pain

PTSD

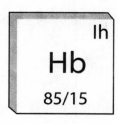

Growing: Moderate

Flowering: 65 - 70 Days

Description: Headband is an Indica dominant strain. This plant tends to grow small-medium height. We would suggest topping two to three times during the vegetative stage.

You can find out more about topping your plants by visiting:

http://professorgrow.com/2010/09/21/mmj-corner-topping-and-cropping-to-increase-your-yield/

This is a good plant for a small grow room. Three plants would do well in a smaller growing area. Keep in mind that it does have a little longer flowering period than most Indicas.

*The *__Past Medicinal Uses__* information in this book is NOT intended to replace the advice of your licensed medical practitioner nor is it intended to diagnose, treat, cure or prevent any disease. It is merely a listing of some historical uses for this particular strain. Contact your licensed medical professional for advice on using various strains for your ailments.

Island Sweet Skunk

Lineage: BC Sweet Pink Grapefruit X Big Skunk #1

Genetics: 70% (S) 30% (I)

THC Content: 15% — 20%

Past Medicinal Uses*:

Appetite Stimulant

Chemotherapy

Epilepsy

Fatigue

Fibromyalgia

Glaucoma

Headaches

Mood Elevation

MS

Nausea

Nerve Pain

RSD (Reflex Sympathetic Dystrophy)

```
        Sh
Iss
   70/30
```

Growing: Moderate

Flowering: 50 - 55 Days

Description: Island Sweet Skunk is a Sativa dominant strain. This plant tends to grow tall. We would suggest topping three to four times during vegetative stage.

You can find out more about topping your plants by visiting:

http://professorgrow.com/2010/09/21/mmj-corner-topping-and-cropping-to-increase-your-yield/

This plant will need a little more room to grow. When putting in to your grow room, keep this in mind, especially if you have a small grow room. We suggest you only grow two plants because of height. The nice thing is that it has a shorter flowering time than most Sativas.

*The **_Past Medicinal Uses_** information in this book is NOT intended to replace the advice of your licensed medical practitioner nor is it intended to diagnose, treat, cure or prevent any disease. It is merely a listing of some historical uses for this particular strain. Contact your licensed medical professional for advice on using various strains for your ailments.

<u>Jack Herer</u>

Lineage: Skunk #1 X NL #5 X Haze

Genetics: 80% (S) 20% (I)

THC Content: 15% — 20%

Awards: 1994 Cannabis Cup 1st Place
            1999 Sativa Cup 1st Place

Past Medicinal Uses*:

ADD
Appetite
Energy
Fibromyalgia
Focus
Nervousness
Pain
Social Anxiety

```
        ┌──────────────┐
        │           Sh │
        │              │
        │   Jh         │
        │   80/20      │
        └──────────────┘
```

Growing: Moderate-Difficult

Flowering: 60 - 70 Days

Description: This is a Sativa dominant strain developed by the legendary Jack Herer. This plant tends to grow to a tall height. It has good natural side branching.

We would suggest topping the plant three to four times to control the height. You can find out more about topping your plants by visiting:

http://professorgrow.com/2010/09/21/mmj-corner-topping-and-cropping-to-increase-your-yield/

This plant can be a little difficult because of it's genetic crosses. Just be patient with the plant. We would not suggest this plant for a small grow room. It would do much better outdoors where it has plenty of room to grow.

*The **_Past Medicinal Uses_** information in this book is NOT intended to replace the advice of your licensed medical practitioner nor is it intended to diagnose, treat, cure or prevent any disease. It is merely a listing of some historical uses for this particular strain. Contact your licensed medical professional for advice on using various strains for your ailments.

<u>Jilly Bean</u>

Lineage: UKN Orange Skunk X Romulan X Cindy 99

Genetics: 70% (I) 30% (S)

THC Content: 12% — 18%

Past Medicinal Uses*:

Anxiety

Appetite Stimulation

Depression

Migraines

Nausea

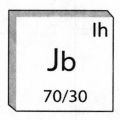

Growing: Easy-Moderate

Flowering: 56 - 63 Days

Description: Jilly Bean is an Indica dominant strain. (Note: We have seen it referenced as a Sativa dominant in some places, and we have seen Jilly Bean plants that looked more Sativa in their leaves and structure. Most sources referred to it as an Indica dominant.) This plant tends to grow small-medium height.

We would suggest topping three to four times during the vegetative stage, to let the plant bush out a little more and create more bud sites. You can find out more about topping your plants by visiting:

http://professorgrow.com/2010/09/21/mmj-corner-topping-and-cropping-to-increase-your-yield/

This plant is ideal for the small grow room. With heavy topping three plants will do well in a small grow room.

*The _**Past Medicinal Uses**_ information in this book is NOT intended to replace the advice of your licensed medical practitioner nor is it intended to diagnose, treat, cure or prevent any disease. It is merely a listing of some historical uses for this particular strain. Contact your licensed medical professional for advice on using various strains for your ailments.

Juicy Fruit

Lineage: Afghani Landrace X Thai Landrace

Genetics: 75% (I) 25% (S)

THC Content: 15% — 20%

Past Medicinal Uses*:

Anti-Anxiety

Energy

Inspiration

Mild Body Pain Relief

Mood Elevation

Motivation

Ocular Attention

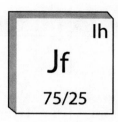

Growing: Easy-Moderate

Flowering: 56 - 63 Days

Description: This is an Indica dominant strain. This plant tends to grow small-medium height.

We would suggest topping three to four times during the vegetative stage to let the plant bush out a little more and create more bud sites. You can find out more about topping your plants by visiting:

http://professorgrow.com/2010/09/21/mmj-corner-topping-and-cropping-to-increase-your-yield/

This plant is ideal for the small grow room. With heavy topping three plants will do well in a small grow room.

*The **_Past Medicinal Uses_** information in this book is NOT intended to replace the advice of your licensed medical practitioner nor is it intended to diagnose, treat, cure or prevent any disease. It is merely a listing of some historical uses for this particular strain. Contact your licensed medical professional for advice on using various strains for your ailments.

LA Confidential

Lineage: O.G. LA Affie X Afghani

Genetics: 100% (I)

THC Content: 15% — 20%

Awards: 2004 Indica Cup 3rd Place
2005 Indica Cup 2nd Place

Past Medicinal Uses*:

ADD
ADHD
Anxiety
Appetite Stimulation
Arthritis
Chronic Pain
Gastrointestinal Disorder
Insomnia
MS
Pain Relief

Lc

I

100

Growing: Easy

Flowering: 45 - 56 Days

Description: This is a pure Indica strain. It tends to grow to a small to medium height. It also has nice side branching, creating multiple bud sites.

We would NOT suggest topping because LA Confidential already has good natural side branching.

This is a great plant for the small grow room. Three plants will do well in a small grow room.

This is a nice plant for a beginner to grow, as it doesn't get too big, doesn't need topping and has a fairly short flowering period.

*The **_Past Medicinal Uses_** information in this book is NOT intended to replace the advice of your licensed medical practitioner nor is it intended to diagnose, treat, cure or prevent any disease. It is merely a listing of some historical uses for this particular strain. Contact your licensed medical professional for advice on using various strains for your ailments.

Lavender Kush

Lineage: Super Skunk X Big Skunk Korean X Afghani/
Hawaiian

Genetics: 80% (I) 20% (S)

THC Content: 15% — 18%

Awards: 2005 Indica Cup 1st Place

Past Medicinal Uses*:

Anxiety

Appetite

Bipolar Disorder

Insomnia

Migraines

Nausea

Pain Relief

PTSD

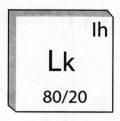

Growing: Easy

Flowering: 53 - 63 Days

Description: Lavender Kush is an Indica dominant strain. This plant tends to grow to a medium height.

We would suggest topping two to three times during the vegetative stage. This will help keep the plant at a good, manageable height and increase the number of bud sites. You can find out more about topping your plants by visiting:

http://professorgrow.com/2010/09/21/mmj-corner-topping-and-cropping-to-increase-your-yield/

Three plants will do well in a small grow room.

*The ***Past Medicinal Uses*** information in this book is NOT intended to replace the advice of your licensed medical practitioner nor is it intended to diagnose, treat, cure or prevent any disease. It is merely a listing of some historical uses for this particular strain. Contact your licensed medical professional for advice on using various strains for your ailments.

Lemon Skunk

Lineage: Skunk #1 X Citral

Genetics: 60% (S) 40% (I)

THC Content: 18% — 22%

Past Medicinal Uses*:

ADHD

Appetite

Autism

Cancer

Epilepsy

Insomnia

Muscle Pain

Seizures

Ls Sh
60/40

Growing: Moderate

Flowering: 50 - 56 Days

Description: Lemon Skunk is a Sativa dominant strain. This plant tends to grow to a medium-tall height.

We would suggest topping three to four times during vegetative stage. This will help keep the plant from getting too tall. You can find out more about topping your plants by visiting:

http://professorgrow.com/2010/09/21/mmj-corner-topping-and-cropping-to-increase-your-yield/

This plant needs a little more room to grow. When putting in to your grow room keep this in mind, especially if you have a small grow room. We suggest you only grow two plants unless you have a big grow area.

*The **_Past Medicinal Uses_** information in this book is NOT intended to replace the advice of your licensed medical practitioner nor is it intended to diagnose, treat, cure or prevent any disease. It is merely a listing of some historical uses for this particular strain. Contact your licensed medical professional for advice on using various strains for your ailments.

<u>Mango Haze</u>

Lineage: NL #5/ Skunk X Haze

Genetics: 50% (S) 50% (I)

THC Content: 15% — 20%

Past Medicinal Uses*:

Anxiety

Depression

Eating Disorders

Inflammation

Migraines

Nausea

Pain Relief

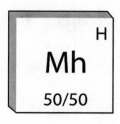

Growing: Moderate-Difficult

Flowering: 50 - 60 Days

Description: This strain is a 50/50 mix of Indica and Sativa. This plant tends to grow to a medium-tall height.

We would suggest topping three to four times during vegetative stage. This will help keep the plant at a good height. You can find out more about topping your plants by visiting:

http://professorgrow.com/2010/09/21/mmj-corner-topping-and-cropping-to-increase-your-yield/

This plant will need a little more room to grow. Keep this in mind if you have a small grow room. We suggest you only grow two plants unless you have a big grow area.

*The _**Past Medicinal Uses**_ information in this book is NOT intended to replace the advice of your licensed medical practitioner nor is it intended to diagnose, treat, cure or prevent any disease. It is merely a listing of some historical uses for this particular strain. Contact your licensed medical professional for advice on using various strains for your ailments.

Master Kush

Lineage: Hindu Kush X Skunk

Genetics: 80% (I) 20% (S)

THC Content: 15% — 18%

Past Medicinal Uses*:

Anxiety

Asthma

Creative Thoughts

Energy

Increased Appetite

Nausea

Relaxation

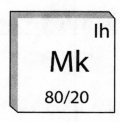

Growing: Easy

Flowering: 63 - 70 Days

Description: This is an Indica dominant strain. This plant tends to grow small.

We would suggest topping two to three times during the vegetative stage to increase the number of bud sites. You can find out more about topping your plants by visiting:

http://professorgrow.com/2010/09/21/mmj-corner-topping-and-cropping-to-increase-your-yield/

This is a good plant for a small grow room. Three plants would do well in a smaller growing area. Just keep in mind that it does have a little longer flowering period than most Indicas.

*The ***Past Medicinal Uses*** information in this book is NOT intended to replace the advice of your licensed medical practitioner nor is it intended to diagnose, treat, cure or prevent any disease. It is merely a listing of some historical uses for this particular strain. Contact your licensed medical professional for advice on using various strains for your ailments.

<u>Maui Wowie</u>

Lineage: Hawaiian Hybrid

Genetics: 70% (S) 30% (I)

THC Content: 8% — 15%

Past Medicinal Uses*:

Arthritis

Asthma

Bipolar Disorder

Depression

Glaucoma

Migraines

PTSD

Tourette's Syndrome

```
        ┌──────────────┐
        │          Sh  │
        │     Mw       │
        │    70/30     │
        └──────────────┘
```

Growing: Moderate-Difficult

Flowering: 60 - 75 Days

Description: Maui Wowie is a Sativa dominant strain. This plant tends to grow to a medium-tall height.

We would suggest topping three to four times during vegetative stage. This will help keep the plant at a good height. You can find out more about topping your plants by visiting:

http://professorgrow.com/2010/09/21/mmj-corner-topping-and-cropping-to-increase-your-yield/

This plant will need a little more room to grow. When putting in to your grow room keep this in mind. If you have a small grow room. We suggest you only grow two plants unless you have a big grow area.

*The **_Past Medicinal Uses_** information in this book is NOT intended to replace the advice of your licensed medical practitioner nor is it intended to diagnose, treat, cure or prevent any disease. It is merely a listing of some historical uses for this particular strain. Contact your licensed medical professional for advice on using various strains for your ailments.

<u>Northern Lights</u>

Lineage: Afghan X Skunk #1 X Haze

Genetics: 95% (I) 5% (S)

THC Content: 15% — 20%

Awards: 1993 Cannabis Cup 2nd Place

Past Medicinal Uses*:

Anxiety

Depression

Hypertension

Insomnia

Lower Back Pain

Nausea

PTSD

```
                    Ih
        NI
        95/5
```

Growing: Easy

Flowering: 45 - 50 Days

Description: Northern Lights is almost a pure Indica strain. This plant tends to grow small- medium height.

We would suggest topping two to three times during the vegetative stage to help produce more budding sites.

You can find out more about topping your plants by visiting:

http://professorgrow.com/2010/09/21/mmj-corner-topping-and-cropping-to-increase-your-yield/

This is a good plant for a small grow room. Three plants would do well in a smaller growing area.

*The _**Past Medicinal Uses**_ information in this book is NOT intended to replace the advice of your licensed medical practitioner nor is it intended to diagnose, treat, cure or prevent any disease. It is merely a listing of some historical uses for this particular strain. Contact your licensed medical professional for advice on using various strains for your ailments.

__NYC Diesel__

Lineage: Sour Diesel X Afghani X Hawaiian

Genetics: 60% (S) 40% (I)

THC Content: 15% — 20%

Awards: 2001 Sativa Cup 3rd Place

2002 Cannabis Cup 2nd Place

2002 Sativa Cup 2nd Place

2003 Cannabis Cup 2nd Place

Past Medicinal Uses*:

Appetite

Depression

Migraines

MS

Stomach Ailments

```
                    Sh
        Nd
        60/40
```

Growing: Moderate

Flowering: 55 - 75 Days

Description: New York City Diesel is a Sativa dominant strain. It
tends to grow to a medium height.

It will have some side branching. We would still suggest you top the
plant two to three times during the vegetative stage to increase side
branching and budding sites. You can find out more about topping
your plants by visiting:

http://professorgrow.com/2010/09/21/mmj-corner-topping-and-
cropping-to-increase-your-yield/

This is a good plant for a small grow room. Two to three plants will do
well in a small space. Keep in mind that it has a longer flowering time.

*The **_Past Medicinal Uses_** information in this book is NOT intended
to replace the advice of your licensed medical practitioner nor is it
intended to diagnose, treat, cure or prevent any disease. It is merely a
listing of some historical uses for this particular strain. Contact your
licensed medical professional for advice on using various strains for
your ailments.

<u>OG Kush</u>

Lineage: Sour Diesel X Chem Dawg

Genetics: 85% (S) 15% (I)

THC Content: 15% — 20%

Past Medicinal Uses*:

Anti-Anxiety

Anti-Depression

Appetite Stimulation

Headaches

Minor Stomach Discomfort

Mood Elevation

Strong Ocular Attention

```
      ┌──────────┐
      │       Sh │
      │   Ok     │
      │  85/15   │
      └──────────┘
```

Growing: Moderate- Difficult

Flowering: 55 - 65 Days

Description: OG Kush is a Sativa dominant strain. It tends to grow medium-tall.

We would suggest topping the plant three to four times during the vegetative stage to give it more side branching. You can find out more about topping your plants by visiting:

http://professorgrow.com/2010/09/21/mmj-corner-topping-and-cropping-to-increase-your-yield/

This plant will need a little more room to grow. When putting in to your grow room keep this in mind. If you have a small grow room. We suggest you only grow two plants because of height, and its potential to take up space.

*The **_Past Medicinal Uses_** information in this book is NOT intended to replace the advice of your licensed medical practitioner nor is it intended to diagnose, treat, cure or prevent any disease. It is merely a listing of some historical uses for this particular strain. Contact your licensed medical professional for advice on using various strains for your ailments.

<u>Purple Haze</u>

Lineage: Purple Haze X Meao Thai

Genetics: 100% (S)

THC Content: 18% — 20%

Past Medicinal Uses*:

ADD

ADHD

Anxiety

Appetite Stimulation

Bipolar Disorder

Cancer

Cramps

Depression

Glaucoma

HIV/AIDS

Insomnia

Joint Pain

Muscle Pain

Muscle Spasms

PMDD

PMS

PTSD

Ph ^S

100

Growing: Difficult

Flowering: 112 - 140 Days

Description: Purple Haze is a pure Sativa strain. This plant will grow very tall. We would suggest topping the plant three to four times during the vegetative stage to keep the height under control. You can find out more about topping your plants by visiting:

http://professorgrow.com/2010/09/21/mmj-corner-topping-and-cropping-to-increase-your-yield/

Also after two-to-two-and-a-half weeks in vegetative state (or when the plant is 18-to-24 inches tall), change the light cycle to the flowering setting. The plant will continue to grow at least 12 to 18 inches in the flowering stage. Purple Haze is not recommended for a small growing area.

*The **_Past Medicinal Uses_** information in this book is NOT intended to replace the advice of your licensed medical practitioner nor is it intended to diagnose, treat, cure or prevent any disease. It is merely a listing of some historical uses for this particular strain. Contact your licensed medical professional for advice on using various strains for your ailments.

Shiva Shanti

Lineage: Northern Lights #5 X Skunk #1

Genetics: 85% (I) 15% (S)

THC Content: 15% — 20%

Awards: 2003 Outdoor Cup 1st Place

Past Medicinal Uses*:

ADHD

Anxiety

Appetite Stimulation

Arthritis

Chronic Pain

Epilepsy

Glaucoma

Insomnia

Migraines

Muscle Spasms

Nausea

Pain Relief

Panic Attacks

PMS

Relaxation

Ih

Ss

85/15

Growing: Easy

Flowering: 44 - 60 Days

Description: Shiva Shanti is an Indica dominant strain. This plant tends to grow small to medium in height.

We would suggest topping two to three times during the vegetative stage to increase side branching and budding sites. You can find out more about topping your plants by visiting:

http://professorgrow.com/2010/09/21/mmj-corner-topping-and-cropping-to-increase-your-yield/

This is a good plant for a small grow room. Three plants would do well in a smaller growing area.

*The ***Past Medicinal Uses*** information in this book is NOT intended to replace the advice of your licensed medical practitioner nor is it intended to diagnose, treat, cure or prevent any disease. It is merely a listing of some historical uses for this particular strain. Contact your licensed medical professional for advice on using various strains for your ailments.

<u>Silver Haze</u>

Lineage: Skunk X NL/ Haze

Genetics: 50% (S) 50% (I)

THC Content: 15% — 18%

Awards: 2005 Cannabis Cup 3rd Place

Past Medicinal Uses*:

Anxiety

Appetite

Epilepsy

Multiple Sclerosis

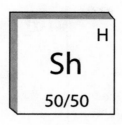

Growing: Easy

Flowering: 56 - 70 Days

Description: Silver Haze is a 50/50 hybrid. This plant tends to grow to a medium-tall height.

We would suggest topping three to four times during vegetative stage. This will help keep the plant at a good height. You can find out more about topping your plants by visiting:

http://professorgrow.com/2010/09/21/mmj-corner-topping-and-cropping-to-increase-your-yield/

This plant needs a little more room to grow. Keep this in mind if you have a small grow room. We suggest you only grow two plants unless you have a big grow area.

*The ***Past Medicinal Uses*** information in this book is NOT intended to replace the advice of your licensed medical practitioner nor is it intended to diagnose, treat, cure or prevent any disease. It is merely a listing of some historical uses for this particular strain. Contact your licensed medical professional for advice on using various strains for your ailments.

Skunk

Lineage: Afghani/ Acapulco Gold X Columbian Gold

Genetics: 60% (I) 40% (S)

THC Content: 10% — 15%

Awards: 1988 Cannabis Cup 1st Place
1989 Indica Cup 2nd Place

Past Medicinal Uses*:

ADD

Alzheimer's Disease

Anxiety

Appetite

Depression

Epilepsy

Insomnia

Nausea

Pain

Tension

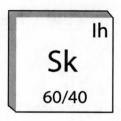

Growing: Easy-Moderate

Flowering: 60 - 74 Days

Description: Skunk is an Indica dominant strain. This plant tends to grow to a medium height.

We would suggest topping two to three times. This will help keep the plant at a good height. You can find out more about topping your plants by visiting:

http://professorgrow.com/2010/09/21/mmj-corner-topping-and-cropping-to-increase-your-yield/

Three plants will do well in a small grow room. Just keep in mind that it does have a little longer flowering period than most Indicas.

*The **_Past Medicinal Uses_** information in this book is NOT intended to replace the advice of your licensed medical practitioner nor is it intended to diagnose, treat, cure or prevent any disease. It is merely a listing of some historical uses for this particular strain. Contact your licensed medical professional for advice on using various strains for your ailments.

Skywalker

Lineage: Mazar X Blueberry

Genetics: 65% (I) 35% (S)

THC Content: 10% — 18%

Past Medicinal Uses*:

Anxiety

Chronic Pain

Insomnia

Muscle Pain

Nausea

Pain

```
        Ih
 Sw
 65/35
```

Growing: Easy

Flowering: 60 - 74 Days

Description: Skywalker is an Indica dominant strain. This plant tends to grow to a medium height.

We would suggest topping two to three times during the vegetative stage. This will help keep the plant at a good height, encourage side branching and increase budding sites. You can find out more about topping your plants by visiting:

http://professorgrow.com/2010/09/21/mmj-corner-topping-and-cropping-to-increase-your-yield/

Three plants should do well in a small grow room if you do your topping two or three times.

*The ***Past Medicinal Uses*** information in this book is NOT intended to replace the advice of your licensed medical practitioner nor is it intended to diagnose, treat, cure or prevent any disease. It is merely a listing of some historical uses for this particular strain. Contact your licensed medical professional for advice on using various strains for your ailments.

<u>Sour Diesel</u>

Lineage: Mexican Sativa X Chemo

Genetics: 90% (S) 10% (I)

THC Content: 12% — 15%

Past Medicinal Uses*:

ADD

ADHD

Anxiety

Depression

Edema

Epilepsy

Fibromyalgia

Migraines

Nausea

Radiculopathy

Sh

Sd

90/10

Growing: Moderate

Flowering: 75 - 80 Days

Description: Sour Diesel is almost a pure Sativa strain. This plant will grow very tall. We would suggest topping the plant three to four times during the vegetative stage to control the height. You can find out more about topping your plants by visiting:

http://professorgrow.com/2010/09/21/mmj-corner-topping-and-cropping-to-increase-your-yield/

After two-to-two-and-a-half weeks in vegetative state (or when the plant is 18-to-24 inches tall), change the light cycle to the flowering setting. The plant will continue to grow at least 12 to 18 inches in the flowering stage.

Sour Diesel is not recommended for a small growing area.

*The ***Past Medicinal Uses*** information in this book is NOT intended to replace the advice of your licensed medical practitioner nor is it intended to diagnose, treat, cure or prevent any disease. It is merely a listing of some historical uses for this particular strain. Contact your licensed medical professional for advice on using various strains for your ailments.

<u>Strawberry Cough</u>

Lineage: Strawberry Fields X Haze

Genetics: 75% (S) 25% (I)

THC Content: 15% — 20%

Past Medicinal Uses*:

ADD

Back Pain

Depression

Gastroenteritis

Joint Pain

Migraines

PTSD

```
                    Sh
         Sc
        75/25
```

Growing: Easy-Moderate

Flowering: 56 - 63 Days

Description: Strawberry Cough is a Sativa dominant strain. It tends to grow to a medium- tall height.

The good thing about this strain is the shorter flowering time for a Sativa dominant strain. And, unlike most Sativas, this strain can be grown in a small grow room.

We suggest two plants. This is because of topping the plants during the vegetative cycle. Topping the plant three to four time will do fine. You can find out more about topping your plants by visiting:

http://professorgrow.com/2010/09/21/mmj-corner-topping-and-cropping-to-increase-your-yield/

*The ___Past Medicinal Uses___ information in this book is NOT intended to replace the advice of your licensed medical practitioner nor is it intended to diagnose, treat, cure or prevent any disease. It is merely a listing of some historical uses for this particular strain. Contact your licensed medical professional for advice on using various strains for your ailments.

<u>Super Lemon Haze</u>

Lineage: Skunk X NL X Haze

Genetics: 75% (S) 25% (I)

THC Content: 18% — 22%

Awards: 2009 Cannabis Cup 1st Place
2009 Sativa Cup 2nd Place
2010 Cannabis Cup 2nd Place

Past Medicinal Uses*:

ADD
ADHD
Appetite Stimulation
Attentive Mind set
Focus
Possible Ocular Relief

```
                    Sh
         Slh
        75/25
```

Growing: Moderate

Flowering: 67 - 85 Days

Description: Super Lemon Haze is a Sativa dominant strain. It tends to grow to a medium-tall height.

We would suggest topping three to four times during vegetative stage. This will help keep the plant at a good height. You can find out more about topping your plants by visiting:

http://professorgrow.com/2010/09/21/mmj-corner-topping-and-cropping-to-increase-your-yield/

 This plant will need a little more room to grow. When putting Super Lemon Haze into your grow room keep this in mind, especially if you have a small grow room. We suggest you only grow two plants unless you have a big grow area.

*The ***Past Medicinal Uses*** information in this book is NOT intended to replace the advice of your licensed medical practitioner nor is it intended to diagnose, treat, cure or prevent any disease. It is merely a listing of some historical uses for this particular strain. Contact your licensed medical professional for advice on using various strains for your ailments.

Super Silver Haze

Lineage: Skunk X NL X Haze

Genetics: 75% (S) 25% (I)

THC Content: 15% — 20%

Awards: 1998 Cannabis Cup 1st Place
1999 Cannabis Cup 1st Place
2007 Cannabis Cup 3rd Place
2008 Cannabis Cup 1st Place

Past Medicinal Uses*:

ADD

ADHD

Anxiety

Appetite

Back Pain

Cramps

Depression

Glaucoma

Joint Pain

Migraines

Muscle Pain

PMDD

PMS

	Sh
Ssh	
75/25	

Growing: Moderate

Flowering: 56 - 70 Days

Description: Super Silver Haze is a Sativa dominant strain. Super Silver Haze tends to grow to a medium-tall height.

We would suggest topping three to four times during vegetative stage. This will help keep the plant at a good height and increase side branching. You can find out more about topping your plants by visiting:

http://professorgrow.com/2010/09/21/mmj-corner-topping-and-cropping-to-increase-your-yield/

This plant needs a little more room to grow. When putting into your grow room keep this in mind, if you have a small grow room. We suggest you only grow two plants unless you have a big growing area.

*The ***Past Medicinal Uses*** information in this book is NOT intended to replace the advice of your licensed medical practitioner nor is it intended to diagnose, treat, cure or prevent any disease. It is merely a listing of some historical uses for this particular strain. Contact your licensed medical professional for advice on using various strains for your ailments.

<u>Train Wreck</u>

Lineage: Afghani X Thai X Mexican/ Columbian

Genetics: 90% (S) 10% (I)

THC Content: 15% — 20%

Past Medicinal Uses*:

Anxiety

Appetite

Arthritis

Diabetic Neuropathy

Insomnia

```
      ┌──────────┐
      │       Sh │
      │   Tw     │
      │  90/10   │
      └──────────┘
```

Growing: Moderate- Difficult

Flowering: 60 - 70 Days

Description: Train Wreck strain is almost a pure Sativa strain. It tends to grow to a medium-tall height.

We would suggest topping three to four times during vegetative stage. This will help keep the plant at a good height and increase side branching. You can find out more about topping your plants by visiting:

http://professorgrow.com/2010/09/21/mmj-corner-topping-and-cropping-to-increase-your-yield/

This plant will need a little more room to grow. When putting in to your grow room keep this in mind, if you have a small grow room. We suggest you only grow two plants unless you have a big grow area.

*The **_Past Medicinal Uses_** information in this book is NOT intended to replace the advice of your licensed medical practitioner nor is it intended to diagnose, treat, cure or prevent any disease. It is merely a listing of some historical uses for this particular strain. Contact your licensed medical professional for advice on using various strains for your ailments.

White Rhino

Lineage: Afghan X Brazilian X South Indian

Genetics: 60 (I) 40% (S)

THC Content: 15% — 20%

Past Medicinal Uses*:

Anti-Inflammatory

Anxiety

Appetite

Chronic Pain

Insomnia

Migraines

MS

Muscle Tension

Nausea

Stomach Pain

Stress

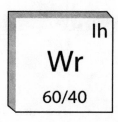

Growing: Easy

Flowering: 60 - 74 Days

Description: White Rhino is an Indica dominant strain. This plant tends to grow small-medium height.

We would suggest topping two to three times during the vegetative stage to increase budding sites. You can find out more about topping your plants by visiting:

http://professorgrow.com/2010/09/21/mmj-corner-topping-and-cropping-to-increase-your-yield/

This is a good plant for a small grow room. Three plants would do well in a smaller growing area. Just keep in mind that White Rhino does have a little longer flowering period than most Indicas.

*The _**Past Medicinal Uses**_ information in this book is NOT intended to replace the advice of your licensed medical practitioner nor is it intended to diagnose, treat, cure or prevent any disease. It is merely a listing of some historical uses for this particular strain. Contact your licensed medical professional for advice on using various strains for your ailments.

White Widow

Lineage: Brazilian X South Indian

Genetics: 60% (S) 40% (I)

THC Content: 15% — 20%

Awards: 1995 Cannabis Cup 1st Place

Past Medicinal Uses*:

Anxiety

Appetite Stimulation

Cachexia

Cancer

Depression

Epilepsy

Fibromyalgia

Glaucoma

Hepatitis C

HIV/AIDS

PTSD

Seizures

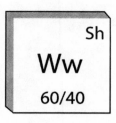

Growing: Easy

Flowering: 60 - 74 Days

Description: White Widow is a Sativa dominant strain. This plant tends to grow small-medium height.

We would suggest topping two to three times during the vegetative stage to increase budding sites. You can find out more about topping your plants by visiting:

http://professorgrow.com/2010/09/21/mmj-corner-topping-and-cropping-to-increase-your-yield/

This is a good plant for a small grow room. Three plants would do well in a smaller growing area.

*The ***_Past Medicinal Uses_*** information in this book is NOT intended to replace the advice of your licensed medical practitioner nor is it intended to diagnose, treat, cure or prevent any disease. It is merely a listing of some historical uses for this particular strain. Contact your licensed medical professional for advice on using various strains for your ailments.

Ailment Index

This Index lists Ailments (alphabetically)along with the cannabis strains that have been used in the past by patients seeking relief for those Ailments.

The information in this index is **NOT** intended to replace the advice of your licensed medical practitioner nor is it intended to diagnose, treat, cure or prevent any disease. It is merely a listing of some historical uses for this particular strain. Contact your licensed medical professional for advice on using various strains of cannabis for your ailments.

As a reference, you can look up an ailment in this index and see what strains have historically been used for that ailment. The Strains are all listed in the Table of Contents (alphabetically).

The authors wish to remind the readers that the use of cannabis for medical purposes is only approved in a limited number of states. We advise you to check your state's laws and regulations and comply with them if you are seeking to be a medical marijuana patient. Use of cannabis for any purpose, including medicinal, remains unlawful under Federal laws.

Ailments and Strains

As a reference, you can look up an ailment in this index and see what strains have historically been used for that ailment. The authors make no recommendations regarding the appropriateness of using any cannabis strain for any purpose.

Aches
AK-47
Bubba Kush
Buddha's Sister
Chocolope
Hash Plant
Island Sweet Skunk
OG Kush

ADD
Bubble Berry
Bubble Gum
Buddha's Sister
Durban Poison
G-13 x Haze
Hawaiian Skunk
Headband
Jack Herer
LA Confidential
Purple Haze
Skunk
Sour Diesel
Strawberry Cough
Super Lemon Haze

ADD (cont.)
Super Silver Haze

ADHD
Buddha's Sister
G-13 x Haze
LA Confidential
Lemon Skunk
Purple Haze
Shiva Shanti
Sour Diesel
Super Lemon Haze
Super Silver Haze

AIDS
Afghan Goo (aka Afghooey)
Blueberry
Blue Dream
G-13
Headband
Purple Haze
White Widow

Alcoholism

Afghan Goo (aka Afghooey)

ALS

Buddha's Sister

Alzheimer's Disease

AK-47

Bubble Gum

Skunk

Anorexia

Afghan Goo (aka Afghooey)

Blueberry

Blue Dream

Blue Moonshine

Chocolope

Headband

Anti-Anxiety

Afghan Goo (aka Afghooey)

Big Bud

Blue Moonshine

Blueberry

Bubba Kush

Bubble Gum

Chem Dog (aka Chem

Dawg)

Durban Poison

Flo

G-13 x Haze

Anti-Anxiety (cont.)

Grapefruit

Hash Plant

Hawaiian

Hawaiian Skunk

Jack Herer

Jilly Bean

Juicy Fruit

LA Confidential

Lavender Kush

Mango Haze

Master Kush

Northern Lights

OG Kush

Purple Haze

Shiva Shanti

Silver Haze

Skunk

Skywalker

Sour Diesel

Super Silver Haze

Train Wreck

White Rhino

White Widow

Anti-Depression

Afghan Goo (aka Afghooey)

Afghooey Train Wreck

AK-47

Big Bud

Blue Dream

Anti-Depression (cont.)

Bubble Berry

Bubble Gum

Blue Moonshine

Buddha's Sister

Chocolope

Durban Poison

G-13 x Haze

Grapefruit

Hash Plant

Hawaiian

Hawaiian Skunk

Hawaiian Snow

Headband

Jilly Bean

Mango Haze

Maui Wowie

Northern Lights

NYC Diesel

OG Kush

Purple Haze

Skunk

Sour Diesel

Strawberry Cough

Super Silver Haze

White Widow

Anti-Fatigue

Flo

Island Sweet Skunk

Anti-Inflammatory

Durban Poison

G-13

Hawaiian Snow

Mango Haze

White Rhino

Anticonvulsant

Bubble Gum

Blue Moonshine

G-13 x Haze

Anxiety

Afghan Goo (aka Afghooey)

Big Bud

Blue Moonshine

Blueberry

Bubba Kush

Bubble Gum

Chem Dog (aka Chem Dawg)

Durban Poison

Flo

G-13 x Haze

Grapefruit

Hash Plant

Hawaiian

Hawaiian Skunk

Jack Herer

Jilly Bean

Juicy Fruit

Anxiety (cont.)

LA Confidential

Lavender Kush

Mango Haze

Master Kush

Northern Lights

OG Kush

Purple Haze

Shiva Shanti

Silver Haze

Skunk

Skywalker

Sour Diesel

Super Silver Haze

Train Wreck

White Rhino

White Widow

Appetite Stimulation

Afghan Goo (aka Afghooey)

Afghooey Train Wreck

AK-47

Big Bud

Blue Dream

Blue Moonshine

Bubble Berry

Bubble Gum

Buddha's Sister

Durban Poison

Flo

G-13 x Haze

Appetite Stim (cont.)

Grand Daddy Purple

Grapefruit

Hash Plant

Hawaiian Skunk

Island Sweet Skunk

Jack Herer

Jilly Bean

LA Confidential

Lavender Kush

Lemon Skunk

Master Kush

NYC Diesel

OG Kush

Purple Haze

Shiva Shanti

Silver Haze

Skunk

Super Lemon Haze

Super Silver Haze

Train Wreck

White Rhino

White Widow

Arthritis Pain

Afghan Goo (aka Afghooey)

Blue Dream

Chocolope

G-13

G-13 x Haze

Headband

Arthritis Pain (cont.)

LA Confidential

Maui Wowie

Shiva Shanti

Train Wreck

Asthma

Maui Wowie

Master Kush

Attentive Mind Set

Jack Herer

Super Lemon Haze

Autism

Lemon Skunk

Back Pain

Northern Lights

Strawberry Cough

Super Silver Haze

Bipolar Disorder

AK-47

Hash Plant

Lavender Kush

Maui Wowie

Purple Haze

Body Aches

Buddha's Sister

Cachexia

White Widow

Cancer

Afghan Goo (aka Afghooey)

Blue Dream

Chocolope

Durban Poison

G-13

Headband

Lemon Skunk

Purple Haze

White Widow

Chronic Pain

AK-47

Blueberry

Chocolope

G-13 x Haze

Hash Plant

LA Confidential

Shiva Shanti

Skywalker

White Rhino

Cramps

Afghooey Train Wreck

Purple Haze

Super Silver Haze

Creative Thoughts

Master Kush

Deep Muscle Pain

Chem Dog (aka Chem Dawg)

Depression

Afghan Goo (aka Afghooey)

Afghooey Train Wreck

AK-47

Big Bud

Blue Dream

Bubble Berry

Bubble Gum

Blue Moonshine

Buddha's Sister

Chocolope

Durban Poison

G-13 x Haze

Grapefruit

Hash Plant

Hawaiian

Hawaiian Skunk

Hawaiian Snow

Headband

Jilly Bean

Mango Haze

Maui Wowie

Northern Lights

NYC Diesel

Depression (cont.)

OG Kush

Purple Haze

Skunk

Sour Diesel

Strawberry Cough

Super Silver Haze

White Widow

Diabetic Neuropathy

Train Wreck

Eating Disorders

Banana Kush

Mango Haze

Edema

Sour Diesel

Energy

Flo

Jack Herer

Juicy Fruit

Master Kush

Epilepsy

Afghan Goo (aka Afghooey)

Blue Dream

Bubble Berry

Buddha's Sister

G-13 x Haze

Epilepsy (cont.)

Hawaiian

Headband

Island Sweet Skunk

Lemon Skunk

Shiva Shanti

Silver Haze

Skunk

Sour Diesel

White Widow

Fibromyalgia

Afghooey Train Wreck

Banana Kush

G-13

Island Sweet Skunk

Jack Herer

Sour Diesel

White Widow

Focus

Super Lemon Haze

Jack Herer

Gastroenteritis

Strawberry Cough

Gastrointestinal Issues

Afghan Goo (aka Afghooey)

Blueberry

Blue Dream

Gastrointestinal (cont.)

G-13 x Haze

LA Confidential

Glaucoma

Afghan Goo (aka Afghooey)

Banana Kush

Blue Dream

Bubble Gum

Chem Dog (aka Chem Dawg)

Chocolope

Durban Poison

G-13

Hawaiian

Hawaiian Snow

Headband

Island Sweet Skunk

Maui Wowie

Purple Haze

Shiva Shanti

Super Silver Haze

Headaches

AK-47

Bubba Kush

Chocolope

Hash Plant

Island Sweet Skunk

OG Kush

Hepatitis C

White Widow

HIV/AIDS

Afghan Goo (aka Afghooey)

G-13

Purple Haze

White Widow

Hypertension

Grapefruit

Northern Lights

Inflammation

Durban Poison

G-13

Hawaiian Snow

Mango Haze

White Rhino

Insomnia

Afghan Goo (aka Afghooey)

Banana Kush

Big Bud

Blueberry

Bubble Berry

Bubba Kush

Blue Moonshine

Buddha's Sister

G-13 x Haze

Grapefruit

Insomnia (cont.)

Grand Daddy Purple

Hawaiian Skunk

LA Confidential

Lavender Kush

Lemon Skunk

Northern Lights

Purple Haze

Shiva Shanti

Skunk

Skywalker

Train Wreck

White Rhino

Inspiration

Juicy Fruit

Joint Pain

Afghooey Train Wreck

Banana Kush

Chem Dog (aka Chem Dawg)

Durban Poison

G-13

Grand Daddy Purple

Hawaiian Snow

Purple Haze

Strawberry Cough

Super Silver Haze

Lou Gehrig's Disease

Buddha's Sister

Migraines

Afghan Goo (aka Afghooey)
Afghooey Train Wreck
Big Bud
Bubble Berry
Chocolope
Durban Poison
G-13 x Haze
Grand Daddy Purple
Hash Plant
Hawaiian Skunk
Hawaiian Snow
Headband
Jilly Bean
Lavender Kush
Mango Haze
Maui Wowie
NYC Diesel
Shiva Shanti
Sour Diesel
Strawberry Cough
Super Silver Haze
White Rhino

Mood Elevation

Chem Dog (aka Chem Dawg)
Flo
Hawaiian
Island Sweet Skunk
Juicy Fruit
OG Kush

Motivation

Juicy Fruit

Movement Disorders

Chem Dog (aka Chem Dawg)

MS

Afghan Goo (aka Afghooey)
Banana Kush
Big Bud
Blue Dream
Bubble Gum
Durban Poison
G-13
Headband
Island Sweet Skunk
LA Confidential
NYC Diesel
Purple Haze
Shiva Shanti
Silver Haze
Super Silver Haze
White Rhino

Multiple Sclerosis

Afghan Goo (aka Afghooey)
Banana Kush
Big Bud
Blue Dream
Bubble Gum
Durban Poison

Multiple Sclerosis (cont.)

G-13

Headband

Island Sweet Skunk

LA Confidential

NYC Diesel

Purple Haze

Shiva Shanti

Silver Haze

Super Silver Haze

White Rhino

Muscle Pain

Afghan Goo (aka Afghooey)

Afghooey Train Wreck

Banana Kush

Blueberry

Blue Dream

Bubble Berry

Chem Dog (aka Chem Dawg)

Durban Poison

Flo

G-13

Headband

Lemon Skunk

Purple Haze

Shiva Shanti

Skywalker

Super Silver Haze

White Rhino

Muscle Spasms

Afghan Goo (aka Afghooey)

Banana Kush

Blue Dream

Bubble Gum

G-13

Headband

Purple Haze

Shiva Shanti

Muscle Tension

Bubble Berry

Flo

White Rhino

Nausea

Afghan Goo (aka Afghooey)

Afghooey Train Wreck

AK-47

Banana Kush

Big Bud

Blueberry

Blue Dream

Bubble Gum

Blue Moonshine

Buddha's Sister

Chem Dog (aka Chem Dawg)

Chocolope

Durban Poison

G-13

Grand Daddy Purple

Nausea (cont.)

Hash Plant
Hawaiian Snow
Headband
Island Sweet Skunk
Jilly Bean
Lavender Kush
Mango Haze
Master Kush
Northern Lights
Shiva Shanti
Skunk
Sour Diesel
Skywalker
White Rhino

Nervousness

Hash Plant
Jack Herer

Neuropathic Pain

Durban Poison
G-13

Ocular Attention

Flo
Juicy Fruit
OG Kush

Pain

Afghan Goo (aka Afghooey)
Afghooey Train Wreck

Pain (cont.)

AK-47
Banana Kush
Big Bud
Blue Dream
Blue Moonshine
Blueberry
Bubba Kush
Bubble Berry
Chem Dog (aka Chem
Dawg)
Chocolope
Durban Poison
Flo
G-13
G-13 x Haze
Grand Daddy Purple
Hash Plant
Hawaiian
Hawaiian Skunk
Hawaiian Snow
Headband
Island Sweet Skunk
Jack Herer
Juicy Fruit
LA Confidential
Lavender Kush
Lemon Skunk
Mango Haze
Northern Lights
Purple Haze

Pain (cont.)

Shiva Shanti

Skunk

Skywalker

Strawberry Cough

Super Silver Haze

White Rhino

Panic Attacks

Shiva Shanti

Phantom Limb Pain

Banana Kush

Durban Poison

PMDD

Purple Haze

Super Silver Haze

PMS

Afghan Goo (aka Afghooey)

Purple Haze

Shiva Shanti

Super Silver Haze

Possible Ocular Relief

Grapefruit

Super Lemon Haze

PTSD

Afghan Goo (aka Afghooey)

Blue Dream

PTSD (cont.)

Headband

Lavender Kush

Maui Wowie

Northern Lights

Purple Haze

Strawberry Cough

White Widow

Radiculopathy

Sour Diesel

Relaxation

Flo

Grapefruit

Grand Daddy Purple

Hash Plant

Master Kush

Shiva Shanti

Restless Behaviors

Chem Dog (aka Chem Dawg)

Seizures

Hawaiian

Lemon Skunk

White Widow

Skin Irritation

G-13

Sleep Aid (Insomnia)

Afghan Goo (aka Afghooey)

Banana Kush

Big Bud

Blueberry

Bubble Berry

Bubba Kush

Blue Moonshine

Buddha's Sister

G-13 x Haze

Grapefruit

Grand Daddy Purple

Hawaiian Skunk

LA Confidential

Lavender Kush

Lemon Skunk

Northern Lights

Purple Haze

Shiva Shanti

Skunk

Skywalker

Train Wreck

White Rhino

Social Anxiety

Jack Herer

Soreness

Bubba Kush

Stiff Muscles

Bubba Kush

Stomach Ailments

Big Bud

Bubble Berry

NYC Diesel

OG Kush

White Rhino

Stomach Pain

Big Bud

Bubble Berry

NYC Diesel

OG Kush

White Rhino

Stomach Ulcers

Bubble Berry

Stress

Big Bud

Bubble Berry

Bubble Gum

Blue Moonshine

Hash Plant

Hawaiian Skunk

White Rhino

Strong Ocular Attention

Flo

Strong Ocular Attention (cont.)

Juicy Fruit

OG Kush

Tension

Bubble Berry

Flo

Skunk

White Rhino

Tourette's Syndrome

Big Bud

Maui Wowie

Vomiting (Nausea)

Afghan Goo (aka Afghooey)

Afghooey Train Wreck

AK-47

Banana Kush

Big Bud

Blueberry

Blue Dream

Bubble Gum

Blue Moonshine

Buddha's Sister

Chem Dog (aka Chem Dawg)

Chocolope

Durban Poison

Vomiting (Nausea) (cont.)

G-13

Grand Daddy Purple

Hash Plant

Hawaiian Snow

Headband

Island Sweet Skunk

Jilly Bean

Lavender Kush

Mango Haze

Master Kush

Northern Lights

Shiva Shanti

Skunk

Sour Diesel

Skywalker

White Rhino

Medical Marijuana States

and the Ailments

Covered by Each State

As far as we know, this information is accurate at the time of printing this book. We derived this information from various states' websites and from NORML (National Organization for the Reform of Marijuana Laws).

Because laws and regulations are constantly changing, we cannot guarantee that it is accurate when you read this.

We suggest you check with your state's website for the latest rules. You can also get information about medical use of marijuana from NORML at: http://norml.org/index.cfm?Group_ID=3391

__Alaska__

Patients diagnosed with the following illnesses are afforded legal protection for using medical marijuana within state defined regulations:

Cachexia

Cancer

Chronic Pain

Epilepsy and other disorders characterized by Seizures

Glaucoma

HIV or AIDS

Multiple Sclerosis and other disorders characterized by Muscle Spasticity

Nausea

Other conditions are subject to approval by the Alaska Department of Health and Social Services.

You can find out more about the Medical Marijuana Laws in Alaska and contact the Marijuana Registry by visiting:

http://www.hss.state.ak.us/dph/bvs/marijuana.htm

__Arizona__

Patients diagnosed with the following illnesses are afforded legal protection for using medical marijuana within state defined regulations:

Cancer

Glaucoma

Positive Status for HIV or AIDS

Hepatitis C

Amyotrophic Lateral Sclerosis (Lou Gehrig's Disease)

Crohn's Disease

Agitation of Alzheimer's Disease

Any Chronic or Debilitating medical condition or its treatment that produces one or more of the following:

Cachexia or Wasting Syndrome

Severe or Chronic Pain

Severe Nausea

Seizures, including those characteristic of Epilepsy

Severe or Persistent Muscle Spasms, including those characteristic of Multiple Sclerosis

Persistent Muscle Spasms or Seizures

Severe Nausea or Pain

Other conditions will be subject to approval by the Arizona Department of Health Services.

You can find out more about the Medical Marijuana Laws in Arizona and contact the Medical Marijuana Program by visiting:

http://www.azdhs.gov/prop203/index.htm

<u>California</u>

Patients diagnosed with any Debilitating illness where the medical use of marijuana has been "deemed appropriate and has been recommended by a physician" are afforded legal protection for using medical marijuana within state defined regulations. Conditions typically covered by the law include but are not limited to:

Arthritis

Cachexia

Cancer

Chronic Pain

HIV or AIDS

Epilepsy

Migraine

Multiple Sclerosis

You can find out more about the Medical Marijuana Laws in California and contact the Medical Marijuana Program by visiting:

http://www.cdph.ca.gov/programs/mmp/Pages/Medical%20Marijuana%20Program.aspx

<u>Colorado</u>

Patients diagnosed with the following illnesses are afforded legal protection for using medical marijuana within state defined regulations:

Cachexia

Cancer

Chronic Pain

Chronic nervous system disorders

Epilepsy and other disorders characterized by Seizures

Glaucoma

HIV or AIDS

Multiple Sclerosis

And other disorders characterized by Muscle Spasticity

Nausea

Other conditions are subject to approval by the Colorado Board of Health.

You can find out more about the Medical Marijuana Laws in Colorado and contact the Medical Marijuana Program by visiting:

http://www.cdphe.state.co.us/hs/medicalmarijuana/index.html

District of Columbia

Patients diagnosed with the following illnesses are afforded legal protection for using medical marijuana within the district defined regulations:

HIV or AIDS

Glaucoma

Conditions characterized by Severe and Persistent Muscle Spasms, such as Multiple Sclerosis

Cancer

Or any other condition, as determined by rule making, that is:

"(i) Chronic or long-lasting

"(ii) Debilitating or interferes with the basic functions of life

(iii) A serious medical condition for which the use of medical marijuana is beneficial:

(I) That cannot be effectively treated by any ordinary medical or surgical measure

"(II) For which there is scientific evidence that the use of medical marijuana is likely to be significantly less addictive than the ordinary medical treatment for that condition.

You can find out more about the Medical Marijuana Laws in Washington, DC and contact their regulating agency, the Alcohol, Beverage Regulation Administration by visiting:

http://abra.dc.gov/DC/ABRA/Education+and+Services/
Medical+Marijuana

<u>Hawaii</u>

Patients diagnosed with the following illnesses are afforded legal protection for using medical marijuana within state defined regulations:

Cachexia

Cancer

Chronic Pain

Crohn's Disease

Epilepsy and other disorders characterized by Seizures

Glaucoma

HIV or AIDS

Multiple Sclerosis and other disorders characterized by Muscle Spasticity

Nausea

Other conditions are subject to approval by the Hawaii Department of Health.

You can find out more about the Medical Marijuana Laws in Hawaii by visiting:

http://www.hawaiipolice.com/misc/medical_mj_rules.htm

<u>Maine</u>

Patients diagnosed with the following illnesses are afforded legal protection for using medical marijuana within state defined regulations:

Epilepsy and other disorders characterized by Seizures
Multiple Sclerosis and other disorders characterized by Muscle Spasticity
Nausea or Vomiting as a result of AIDS or Cancer chemotherapy
Cancer
Glaucoma
Positive Status for Human Immunodeficiency Virus (HIV)
Acquired Immune Deficiency Syndrome (AIDS)
Hepatitis C
Amyotrophic Lateral Sclerosis (ALS)
Crohn's Disease
Agitation of Alzheimer's Disease
Nail-Patella Syndrome
Intractable Pain
A Chronic or Debilitating Disease or medical condition or its treatment that produces one or more of the following:
Cachexia or Wasting Syndrome
Severe Nausea
Seizures, including but not limited to those characteristic of Epilepsy
Severe and Persistent Muscle Spasms, including but not limited to those characteristic of Multiple Sclerosis
Any other medical condition or its treatment approved by the department as provided.
You can find out more about the Medical Marijuana Laws in Maine and contact the Marijuana Registry by visiting:

http://www.maine.gov/legis/lawlib/medmarij.html

__Michigan__

Patients diagnosed with the following illnesses are afforded legal protection for using medical marijuana within state defined regulations or the treatment of these conditions.:

Cancer

Glaucoma

Positive Status for Human Immunodeficiency Virus (HIV)

Acquired Immune Deficiency Syndrome (AIDS)

Hepatitis C

Amyotrophic Lateral Sclerosis

Crohn's Disease

Agitation of Alzheimer's Disease

Nail Patella

Chronic or Debilitating Disease or medical condition or treatment of said condition that produces 1 or more of the following:

Cachexia or Wasting Syndrome

Severe and Chronic Pain

Severe Nausea

Seizures, including but not limited to those characteristic of Epilepsy

Severe and Persistent Muscle Spasms, including but not limited to those characteristic of Multiple Sclerosis.

You can find out more about the Medical Marijuana Laws in Michigan and contact the Marijuana Registry by visiting:

http://www.michigan.gov/mdch/0,1607,7-132-27417_51869—,00.html

<u>Montana</u>

Patients diagnosed with the following illnesses are afforded legal protection for using medical marijuana within state defined regulations:

Cachexia or Wasting Syndrome

Severe or Chronic Pain

Severe Nausea

Seizures, including but not limited to those characteristic of Epilepsy

Persistent Muscle Spasms, including but not limited to those characteristic of Multiple Sclerosis

Crohn's Disease

You can find out more about the Medical Marijuana Laws in Montana and contact the Marijuana Registry by visiting:

http://www.dphhs.mt.gov/medicalmarijuana/

<u>Nevada</u>

Patients diagnosed with the following illnesses are afforded legal protection for using medical marijuana within state defined regulations:

AIDS

Cancer

Glaucoma

And any medical condition or treatment to a medical condition that produces Cachexia

Persistent Muscle Spasms

Seizures

Severe Nausea or Pain

Other conditions are subject to approval by the health division of the State Department of Human Resources.

You can find out more about the Medical Marijuana Laws in Nevada and contact the Marijuana Registry by visiting:

http://health.nv.gov/MedicalMarijuana.htm

New Jersey

Governor Jon Corzine signed the New Jersey Compassionate Use Medical Marijuana Act into law on January 18, 2010. Lawmakers amended the legislation at the behest of Republican Gov. Chris Christie to delay the enactment of the law until October 1, 2010. The law mandates the state to promulgate rules governing the distribution of medical cannabis to state-authorized patients. These rules shall address the creation of up to six state-licensed "alternative treatment centers." Patients diagnosed with the following illnesses are afforded legal protection under this act:

Cancer

Glaucoma

Seizure and/or Spasticity disorders (including Epilepsy)

Lou Gehrig's Disease

Multiple Sclerosis

Muscular dystrophy

HIV/AIDS

Inflammatory bowel Disease (including Crohn's Disease)

Any terminal illness if a doctor has determined the patient will die within a year.

You can find out more about the Medical Marijuana Laws in New Jersey and contact the Marijuana Registry by visiting:

http://www.state.nj.us/health/med_marijuana.shtml

New Mexico

Patients registered with the State Department of Health and who are diagnosed with the following illnesses are afforded legal protection for using medical marijuana within state defined regulations:

Arthritis

Severe Chronic Pain

Painful Peripheral Neuropathy

Intractable Nausea/Vomiting

Severe Anorexia/Cachexia

Hepatitis C infection currently receiving antiviral treatment

Crohn's Disease

Post-Traumatic Stress Disorder (PTSD)

Amyotrophic Lateral Sclerosis (ALS or Lou Gehrig's Disease)

Cancer

Glaucoma

Multiple Sclerosis

Damage to the nervous tissue of the spinal cord with Intractable Spasticity

Epilepsy

HIV/AIDS

Hospice patients

You can find out more about the Medical Marijuana Laws in New Mexico and contact the Marijuana Registry by visiting:

http://www.health.state.nm.us/idb/medical_cannabis.shtml

<u>Oregon</u>

Patients diagnosed with the following illnesses are afforded legal protection for using medical marijuana within state defined regulations:

Cachexia

Cancer

Chronic Pain

Epilepsy and other disorders characterized by Seizures

Glaucoma

HIV or AIDS

Multiple Sclerosis and other disorders characterized by Muscle Spasticity

Agitation due to Alzheimer's Disease

Nausea

Other conditions are subject to approval by the Health Division of the Oregon Department of Human Resources.

You can find out more about the Medical Marijuana Laws in Oregon and contact the Marijuana Registry by visiting:

http://www.oregon.gov/DHS/ph/ommp/index.shtml

Rhode Island

Patients diagnosed with the following illnesses are afforded legal protection under this act:

Cachexia

Cancer

Glaucoma

Hepatitis C

Severe, Debilitating, Chronic Pain

Severe Nausea

Seizures, including but not limited to, those characteristic of Epilepsy

Severe and Persistent Muscle Spasms, including but not limited to, those characteristic of:

Multiple Sclerosis or Crohn's Disease

Agitation of Alzheimer's Disease

Other conditions are subject to approval by the Rhode Island Department of Health.

You can find out more about the Medical Marijuana Laws in Rhode Island and contact the Marijuana Registry by visiting:

http://www.health.ri.gov/healthcare/medicalmarijuana/

__Vermont__

Patients diagnosed with the following illnesses are afforded legal protection for using medical marijuana within state defined regulations:

HIV or AIDS

Cancer

Multiple Sclerosis

Positive Status for Human Immunodeficiency Virus (HIV)

Acquired Immune Deficiency Syndrome (AIDS)

or the treatment of these conditions, if the Disease or the treatment

results in Severe, Persistent, and Intractable symptoms

A Disease, medical condition, or its treatment that is Chronic, Debilitating, and produces Severe, Persistent, and one or more of the following Intractable symptoms:

Cachexia or Wasting Syndrome

Severe Pain

Severe Nausea

Seizures."

You can find out more about the Medical Marijuana Laws in Vermont and contact the Marijuana Registry by visiting:

http://www.dps.state.vt.us/cjs/marijuana.htm

<u>Washington</u>

Patients diagnosed with the following illnesses are afforded legal protection for using medical marijuana within state defined regulations:

Cachexia

Cancer

HIV or AIDS

Epilepsy

Glaucoma

Intractable Pain (defined as Pain unrelieved by standard treatment or medications)

Multiple Sclerosis

Crohn's Disease

Hepatitis C
Any "Diseases, including Anorexia, which results in Nausea, Vomiting, Wasting, Appetite Loss, Cramping, Seizures

Muscle Spasms, and/or Spasticity, when these symptoms are unrelieved by standard treatments or medications."

You can find out more about the Medical Marijuana Laws in Washington state and contact the Marijuana Registry by visiting:

http://www.doh.wa.gov/hsqa/medical-marijuana/

Cannabis Analysis Labs

CannabAnalysis Laboratories

Missoula, MT

Phone: 406-531-6726

www.cannabanalysis.com

Contact: Rose Habib

rose@cannabanalysis.com

CW Analytical Laboratories

Oakland, CA

Phone: 510-545-6984

www.cwanalytical.com

lab@cwanalytical.com

Full Spectrum Labs

4260 Kearney Street

Denver, CO 80216

Phone: 720-335-5227

www.fullspectrumlabs.com

info@fullspectrumlabs.com

help@fullspectrumlabs.com

Montana Botanical Analysis, LLC

300 N Willson, Suite 105A

Bozeman, MT 59715

Phone: 208-310-0552

www.montanabotanicalanaylysis.com

info@montanabotanicalanaylysis.com

Steep Hill Labs, Inc.

1530 East 12th Street

Oakland, CA 94606

Phone: 510-698-4446

Fax: 510-842-8720

www.steephilllab.com

info@steephilllab.com

As of this writing, these are the five labs in the United States that do chemical analysis of cannabis. As we update this book, we will add more labs as they become available.

NOTE: It is unlawful to send cannabis through the mail or via a private shipping service (such as FEDEX or UPS) to a testing lab. You will have to carry your samples in for testing.

If you have questions about testing your medical marijuana, please contact one of the labs listed here, or if you know of another analysis lab that tests cannabis, contact them.

138

NOTES:

NOTES:

CPSIA information can be obtained at www.ICGtesting.com
Printed in the USA
LVOW111402140212

268659LV00001B/43/P